# The
# San Francisco
# Weight-Loss
# Method

# The San Francisco Weight-Loss Method

24 Minutes a Day to Permanent THIN

Dr. David A. Schoenstadt

Arthur Fields Books, Inc.     New York     1975

Published simultaneously in Canada by Clarke, Irwin & Company Limited, Toronto and Vancouver
ISBN: 0-525-63009-0
LCC: 73-78969
Designed by The Etheredges

To Julie, Randi and Stacey

# Contents

# Acknowledgments

There are several people without whom this book would never have been possible. I am particularly grateful to Harvey Glasser, who helped develop and run this weight-loss program; John O'Neil, who always said the right word at the right time; Herb and Mimi Seidman, who gave me much more than the recipes in this book; and Ray Simons, who worked so hard on the programmed teaching manuals.

And special thanks to two thousand formerly fat people who sweated, went hungry, and eventually proved that this program works.

# The
# San Francisco
# Weight-Loss
# Method

# Why I Know All About Fat

I'll never forget my med-school roommate, Tom. Each year when I receive his Christmas card, the same picture flashes to mind. I see him stretched out on his bed in our tiny dorm room—all six feet and 165 pounds of him—jamming milk shakes and hot dogs into his mouth. At that point in my life I weighed in at 220, and as Tom ate, I would sit on my bed sipping a glass of water. Tom would say, "You ought to have more pride in your appearance, Dave. You know, really *do* something about your weight—I mean, start eating like a normal person."

Later, Tom would excuse himself to go off on a date.

1

I would sit down at my desk to study, but before long I'd end up thinking about my body, asking myself why, why was I so fat? Tom was the one who gorged himself every night, while I was practically starving. How did fat happen to *me*?

Though my fellow medical students would never have believed it, I'd been captain of our high school football team. My coach thought I might even make a career of it, if only I could put on some weight. If I could gain just 6 pounds, he said, and get up to 175, I'd have a good chance of making the all-Chicago team.

I stuffed myself with milk shakes, pastries, fried chicken, french fries. I ate whole pizzas for after-school snacks, but I *couldn't gain even one pound*. I was frustrated, I was miserable, and I never made the connection: unless I was willing to discontinue my daily workouts on the football field, I would never be able to put on a pound.

I didn't make the all-Chicago team, but it didn't really matter—in college I forgot about sports and started concentrating on such sedentary pursuits as medicine and women. And sure enough, my first year off the squad I acquired an enormous talent for gaining weight. I *still* didn't make the connection between weight control and exercise, though, and three years later, when I entered medical school, I carried 45 more pounds than when I'd picked up my high school diploma.

At med school I went on my first diet. I began by cutting out breakfast, and ultimately I cut out lunch too.

Even on one meal a day I continued to gain and soon passed the 220 mark on my scale. (I hated that scale more than I can say, but it became the center of my life. I could never resist the morbid satisfaction of getting on, staring miserably at the indicator, and spending the rest of the day in depression.)

When I hit 220, roommate Tom appointed himself my diet doctor, though he had a few years left before taking the Hippocratic oath. In one of our medical journals he'd read that cutting down to only one meal a day actually *increased* a body's tendency to gain weight. The authors of the article theorized that food could be absorbed better, and weight gain avoided, if one ate six tiny meals a day. Happy to take Tom's advice, I went back to breakfast, lunch, and dinner, and added midmorning, evening, and bedtime snacks, which I'd never indulged in before. Tom was confident that his plan would work. His girl friend had a lovely roommate, and in no time at all, he assured me, we would be a handsome foursome and have lots of laughs together.

But the only laugh to be had was on *me*. In no time at all I'd reached 230. My lab coats wouldn't close, the waist buttons popped on my shirts, I had to buy new pants. And the lovely homecoming queen went home with someone else. I went back to one meal a day and my weight fell back to 210, where it remained for three years.

In 1959, my fourth year of med school, I was still eating one meal a day. That was the year I took Nutrition

Clinic. There I learned that the average person requires 15 calories per pound to maintain body weight. Since I weighed 210, I could eat 3,150 calories a day without gaining weight. And if I could cut down to only 1,000 calories, the deficit of 2,150 calories would enable me to lose 4 or 5 pounds per week.

To say that I was scrupulous in sticking to a 1,000-calorie limit hardly does me justice. I counted every lettuce leaf. Even so, I was eating more than I ever had before. I stayed on the 1,000-calorie diet for twenty-six excruciating weeks. By Nutrition Clinic calculations, I should have weighed 80 pounds! Needless to say, I didn't, but I *had* lost 40 pounds. Two months away from graduation, I was a gorgeous 170. And, having reached the perfect weight, I promptly went off the diet.

I spent my first day of freedom telling people how terrific I felt. Frankly, I didn't really feel that good. I missed certain things that I hadn't eaten for the last six months. I missed pizza. I missed Chinese food and a very special place on Fifty-fifth street near the University of Chicago that served french-fried doughnuts and barbecued ribs.

I went to my very favorite pizzeria and ordered the jumbo combination special.

I knew very well that a cheese, sausage, green-pepper, anchovy, and whatever pizza had to be at least 3,500 calories, and I knew equally well from Nutrition Clinic that 3,500 calories meant 1 pound of fat. However,

I had just lost 40 pounds, and gaining one pound back seemed a modest price to pay for this well-deserved gift to myself.

The pizza was delicious. The anchovies made me thirsty, though, and I had a few beers. Back at the dorm I stopped at the fountain in the lobby for a long drink of ice-cold water.

When I got up to my room I weighed myself. The scale said 178 pounds—178! I had gained 8 pounds in one evening.

I was shocked, but it was too late to put on the brakes. I had tasted pizza after a long abstinence and now there was no stopping me. The next night I did my act at a Chinese restaurant; the next morning I weighed 182 pounds. It had taken me six months to lose 40 pounds and two meals to put back 12.

Three weeks later I was back to 210 pounds. I had decided I would go through life fat. One thing bothered me, though. I was about to begin my internship in southern California, the land of sand and surf, and I really wanted to be a handsome, bronzed specimen in a tiny bathing suit gazing at the Pacific Ocean with my arm around a long-haired, long-legged California maiden. Therefore, one month before I graduated from medical school, I decided I would not eat again until I got to California.

And so, by hovering just above the bounds of strict starvation, I weighed in at 185 pounds, not really looking too bad. For a bronzed California god, I was a little bulgy, but I had youth on my side. I was able to carry it off.

On November 3, 1960, I was married. A month later I was back to 210. Obesity and I would spend ten more years together.

After my internship I moved to Palo Alto to take specialty training. I was always easy to find; doctors just asked for the fat resident. Lounging around the coffee machine one day, a few other residents, some nurses, and I got onto the silly subject of age-guessing. Six people placed me between thirty-five and thirty-nine. When I said I was twenty-five, there was dead silence. "Incredible," someone said. The nurse who'd guessed thirty-nine tried to apologize by saying, "Well, it's just that you look so . . . mature!"

Time to go on a diet. Again. In rapid succession, I discovered the spinach diet, the egg diet, the water diet, and a multitude of others. But I was never really able to get below 195 pounds again.

I began to come home from work exhausted. After dinner I'd sit down in front of the television and fall asleep. At twenty-seven I had settled comfortably into old age. Each morning I had to drag myself out of bed. I went to the hospital, worked two or three hours before I felt really awake and alert, and by mid-afternoon I was exhausted again. When I got home, I went to sleep on the couch. If friends called to invite us out, I usually found some reason to refuse. Or I would try to convince them to come to my house so that I wouldn't have to get up, find my shoes, find

6

my sports coat, drag myself out. If they did come to my house, I tried to be pleasant company, while secretly hoping that they would leave before 10:30 P.M., because it was hard for me to stay awake later than that.

After ten miserable years of fat, when I'd reached 230 pounds, I found the fad diet that worked best for me, the Doctor's Quick Weight Loss Diet. I didn't know it then, but this diet was particularly well suited to me because my metabolism handles carbohydrates particularly poorly.

I lost weight rapidly on this high-protein, no-carbohydrate diet: 30 pounds the first month, 10 the second month, and another 10 the third month. After three months of restricting myself to meat, fish, poultry, cottage cheese, and eggs, I was down to 180 pounds.

I was so sick of walking into a restaurant and ordering the Diet Special (hamburger and cottage cheese), that I began to hate restaurants. Food lost all interest for me.

But no one can forget the eating habits of a lifetime. So, at the end of the three months, I had my first sandwich. And began my climb back to 230 pounds. At 195 pounds, my double chin reappeared and, alarmed, I tried to go back to the high-protein, no-carbohydrate diet. But I couldn't do it, even for a day. Despite the compliments of friends and family, despite the pride I felt when I looked at myself in the mirror, despite feeling better than I had for five or six years, I could not make it through a day without sneaking *some* carbohydrate. I couldn't believe my lack of control, but I had no willpower. None.

The scale was moving rapidly up again and I could do nothing but stand back and watch my new slimness disappear into a great mountain of fat.

Then I had a strange piece of good luck.

I was on obstetrical call when I suddenly became dizzy. I took my pulse; it was very erratic. I went to surgery and attached myself to the heart monitor. There were a few normal beats, then the oscilloscope recorded a dangerously ragged graph. This was the kind of rhythm that precedes cardiac arrest.

One moment I was a thirty-five-year-old physician, caring for the sick, preparing for a full day of operations. The next moment I was flat on my back, wires attached to my chest, an intravenous dripping a heart-relaxing drug into my system, watching my life go by in the green line of an oscilloscope.

I was terrified. During the three days I lay staring at the monitor, I decided I wasn't ready to leave this life. I wanted to go on living. I didn't want to leave my wife. I wanted to see my children grow up.

I left the hospital determined to do whatever was necessary to strengthen my heart. After reading every paper I could find on heart-attack prevention, I settled on Kenneth Cooper's *Aerobics* (M. Evans, 1968) as the most sensible.

Dr. Cooper believes that a person needs to be active for a measured amount of time over a measured distance. In that fixed period of exercise time, the prolonged strain taxes one's breathing, muscles, and blood circulation—and the strain *strengthens* the whole system.

I started on a very gradual, very minimal program of riding a stationary bicycle one mile in ten minutes every day. I hated it. It made me tired and sweaty, and after one week I didn't feel any stronger. I worried about my weak heart for two weeks, then tried again. A week later I gave up for the second time. Then I felt guilty about being a quitter, so I tried a third time, only to quit after just three days.

Despite my intense fear of heart attack and my firm belief that only a program of exercise could save my life, I was unable to get started. Finally my fear of dying proved stronger than my resistance to exertion. On my fourth try I stuck with it for several weeks. Exercise wasn't so bad after all!

After several weeks of my own gentle schedule, I began trying to do a little more pedaling each time I got on my stationary bike. After seven weeks of that, I began to feel so energetic and happy that I found myself actually looking forward to my living-room bicycle ride.

Fifteen weeks after I had begun the bicycling program, I achieved a minimum level of physical fitness. I was also down to 182 pounds!

I couldn't understand how I'd lost the weight. The harder I bicycled, the more my appetite increased. Soon I was eating more than I had when I weighed 230 pounds, but now my weight remained between 175 and 182.

My weight wasn't the only thing that changed. My whole style of life was altered. Instead of getting up tired after eight or nine hours' sleep, I found myself going to bed late and feeling well rested the next morning. I no longer fell asleep in front of the television. In fact, I began to spend a lot less time watching the tube. I rediscovered my friends and, instead of napping away my free time at the hospital, started meeting new people. A few years before, when I was so fat that bending over made me dizzy, I had put my skis in storage. Now I took them out and discovered that I could tighten the bindings with ease. Back on the slopes, I no longer grew painfully short of breath at 7,000 or 8,000 feet. Corny as it may sound, I began to feel as vigorous as a teen-ager again. Best of all, my heart no longer showed any signs of abnormal rhythm.

Obviously something had changed in my body. Not only was I feeling terrific but I was able to eat a good deal of food without gaining weight. Excited by my discovery, I began proselytizing among my friends and associates at the hospital. A close friend, Dr. Harvey Glasser, witnessed the changes in my life and decided his own obese patients would benefit from a gentle exercise program. Together we worked out the details of the health program you will read about in this book.

We began by considering the psychology of dieters. Most people require instant gratification. A diet that de-livers a 15-pound weight loss the first week—even if it *is* mostly water—exhilarates the dieter and renews his or her determination. From then on, he or she will probably lose only 1 or 2 pounds a week, at most, but the momentum of that first big loss will hold the fat person to the diet for weeks afterward.

In contrast, Dr. Glasser and I were faced with the opposite situation: for people on our program, the first week would be the worst. Like me, they would find themselves tired and sweaty, but not feeling significantly better, despite all their effort. After fifteen weeks I was addicted to the good feelings exercise gave me, but how many dieters would be willing to wait nearly four months for results?

Based on these considerations, the outline of our program began to emerge. Obviously we were going to have to devise a beginning program short enough to encourage participation, yet long enough to give our patients a taste of the benefits of the plan. Once they felt their body chemistry *begin* to change, once they began to wake up feeling energetic, then we'd have them hooked. We therefore sketched out a tentative program of forty-nine days. In seven weeks many patients would actually achieve physical fitness. Others—like me—would need more work, but after seven weeks they would feel enormously better and would probably stick with the plan until they succeeded.

We also decided to accompany the exercise with a diet. A sensible diet would accelerate weight loss and help people stick out the exercise program. The second advantage of the diet was less obvious but equally important. The diet would introduce, one by one, the seven basic groups into which virtually all foods are divided, based on the amount of protein, fat, and carbohydrate each contains. During the test diet our patients would encounter each group separately and learn which foods their bodies handled well and which poorly. Although physical fitness will make you "calorie-proof," fitness is further away for some people than for others. As I'll explain fully in the next chapter, people who get into shape more slowly ought to test their body's responses to various foods—and then *stay away from* bread, fruit, milk, or whatever it is that spells trouble for them, at least until they've achieved physical fitness. The test diet we decided to use ran for six weeks— almost as long as the minimal exercise period we'd agreed on. So we added another week to the diet and came up with a program of forty-nine days. Forty of Dr. Glasser's patients were the first to try it out.

*Without exception,* every patient we worked with lost weight. Even more important, many felt the benefits of exercise so dramatically that they continued their physical activity after the end of the program. To date, fully 50 percent of that original test group has *kept off* the weight they lost.

Those first forty-nine days, however, were critical. Harvey Glasser spent a lot of time encouraging his patients to complete seven weeks of continuous exercise. Later on, my wife did the same with friends of ours who also tried the plan. But once we got people past the forty-nine-day barrier, there was no longer any need for pep talks. They all began to feel the wonderful benefits that I had experienced.

Encouraged by our success with patients and friends, Dr. Glasser and I opened a weight-loss clinic in San Francisco. The plan we used has been modified for this book but is basically the same. Neither of us is associated with any other weight-loss method.

Our hundreds of patients have had fantastic results. Six months, a year, and two or more years later, over half our patients who lost weight rapidly during those first forty-nine days have *kept it off*.

Your first question about our plan probably is: All right, what's the gimmick? Lettuce three times a day for the rest of my life? Is this the praying man's diet, the no-food diet, the sex diet? Do you want to insert a tapeworm into my system, as one diet plan actually proposed?

I have no such magical solution, no elixir. Making love instead of snacking may be pleasant, and a diet that prescribes grapefruit six times a day will be greeted with hurrahs by grapefruit growers—but neither will result in *long-term* weight loss for you. This book is for people who are willing to work at a plan for systematic, *permanent* weight loss.

The ultimate aim of this book is to allow you to give up dieting forever. The forty-nine-day plan thus has its own built-in obsolescence. It is a temporary diet, to be replaced by lifelong slimness and carefree eating.

I have experienced every step, every word, every activity mentioned in this book, and I know the program works. A few years ago I was a fat, stay-at-home, lethargic candidate for cardiac arrest. Many fat people mope through life as I did then, living at less than half the energy level they could attain. Having been there myself, I *know* that this plan will produce a dramatic change—and with far less effort than a starvation diet requires.

If you want to *overcome* your weight problem instead of just bouncing up and down the scale, you will eventually have to follow a program similar to mine. Otherwise, you will spend your lifetime in a constant struggle against fat—a battle in which the odds of your long-term success are less than two in one hundred.

As you can see, there's really no choice.

So let's get started with a trip to my clinic for an examination of your obesity.

# What's Your Secret, Dr. Schoenstadt?

If you live in San Francisco, you might be referred to my clinic by your family doctor because your weight has become a medical problem—pushing you toward a heart attack or diabetes, maybe aggravating your arthritis. Or you might make the decision on your own, because the last time you bought slacks you found you had grown two sizes. Or perhaps you just looked at yourself in the mirror while toweling dry after a shower and didn't like what you saw.

Whatever brings you to our door, most likely you are not sure exactly what to expect. You might think we're

15

running a gym when you look around and see several patients on stationary bicycles. Right away you will have a negative reaction: *Exercise! Forget it!*

But once you are comfortably seated in my office, we won't talk about bicycles. What we'll talk about is *you*. Your body. Your weight-loss goals. I'll ask you to review for me every type of diet you've tried, how much you lost each time and how soon you put the weight back on. Confronted with the data of your own past, you will begin to realize for yourself something I talk about a lot, both at the clinic and in this book: *dieting alone won't work.* Seated in my clinic for the first time (or in your living room, reading this chapter), you probably weigh as much as or more than you did when you bought your first diet book.

If you think back over your own dieting history, you'll realize that you already know that dieting alone won't work. What you may *not* already know are the official statistics: no diet ever produced *permanent* weight loss in more than 2 percent of its followers. No matter how successful a diet is for you, the chances are 98 in 100 that you will be fat again within two years.

This program is offering you much more than a two-year respite from your fat life. Yes, you will lose weight. During the next forty-nine days you will lose up to 30 pounds, maybe more. But what I am really prescribing for you is a health program that you should stick to for the rest of your life. In this book I am going to lay out for you a breaking-in period, during which you will learn basic facts about nutrition and your body. During these forty-nine days you will also ease yourself into an exercise program that *will keep that weight off, not just for two years but for the rest of your life*. And all it takes is twenty-four minutes a day.

We'll begin the program by educating you. You need to know how various kinds of food affect your body. As I mentioned before, carbohydrates are my personal Waterloo, while other people have the same trouble with fats. To find out which foodstuff gives *your* body the most trouble, we'll teach you about the seven groups into which most foods you normally eat are divided. Week One of the plan will be a fairly traditional low-calorie diet. Then in each of the remaining six weeks we'll add a new kind of food. By encountering each food group separately, under test conditions, you will become aware of the effects each group has on both your ability to lose weight and your tendency to gain.

You are also going to learn an exchange system that will enable you to eat the foods you like best—a banana split or a pizza, for example—without triggering a huge weight gain and the beginning of a fast climb back to a fat body. Eat pizza and stay thin? If you aren't familiar with food exchanges, this may sound like so much pie in the sky. Actually it's simple mathematics. And it works.

Now, I'm afraid, I *do* have to talk about exercise. It's unavoidable. Because just as important as the ways you handle food is the way you develop your body. But even though it is one of the most hated words in the vocabulary of health, "exercise" *doesn't* have to mean forty sit-ups before breakfast. Over the next couple of months we will be working out an exercise plan that will fit into your life, not dominate it. Although you do have to make special efforts when you are fat, it's nevertheless essential to any weight-loss program that you keep your life as normal as possible. If the measures you take to lose weight constitute a traumatic interruption of your normal habits, chances are you won't stick with them long. What we are aiming at is an exercise plan that can become an ongoing, permanent part of your life.

Why is the exercise regimen so important? Opponents of exercise are fond of pointing out that jogging burns relatively few calories—a recent study showed that a 220-pound man who jogged a mile and a half in ten minutes would burn only 219 calories; a 119-pound man who covered the same distance would burn almost a hundred calories less. Since you must expend 3,500 calories to lose a single pound of fat, you would have to jog every day for a year to lose 10 pounds! And a more substantial weight loss of, say, 50 pounds would take *five* years.

Whether deliberately or through ignorance, these critics of exercise are missing the point. If burning a few hundred calories were the only reason to exercise, believe me, I wouldn't ask you to do it. Exercise is essential for two other reasons: first, it will change your body's composition; second, it will change your body's chemistry. The net result of these changes? At the same time that you are feeling more energetic than you have in years, you will also greatly increase the number of calories you can eat without gaining weight. And if you make a place in your life for twenty-four minutes of daily exercise, you will eventually be able to eat normally while maintaining your ideal weight. To understand how this miracle-working can take place, you must understand more about your body and how it works.

Your body (and everyone else's) is composed of two basic elements. The first, and probably more familiar to you, is your fat, flabby body mass. I know how you feel about fat. I don't blame you. However, we all need *some* fat to function properly, and women need more than men. Ideally, a man's fat should constitute about 10 to 15 percent of his body weight; a woman's fat should be 15 to 25 percent of hers. Unfortunately, fat people's fat often exceeds 50 percent of their body weight. A 200-pound woman may actually consist of a 90-pound woman dragging around more than 110 pounds of fat. Besides being unsightly, this fat burns very few calories and is practically self-sustaining. You'll soon learn why this is so important.

If this 200-pound woman—let's call her Nancy—were to plan a diet, she would have to calculate how many calories she requires to maintain body weight, and then eat *less* than that. Since she makes four beds, vacuums a thousand square feet of carpet, and washes three sets of dishes a day, Nancy decides that she is "moderately active." Referring to a calorie chart, she sees that a moderately active person requires 15 calories per pound to maintain body weight. Since she weighs 200 pounds, she concludes that she needs 3,000 calories per day to maintain her weight. If Nancy wants to lose 1 pound in a week, she has to eat 3,500 calories less than usual, or 500 calories less per day. Nancy decides that her goal is to lose 3 pounds a week, so she must eat 1,500 calories less per day. She subtracts those 1,500 calories from the 3,000 her body requires for maintenance, and goes on a 1,500-calorie diet. At the end of a week she finds that, instead of losing 3 pounds, she has *gained* weight.

Checking her calculations, she figures that maybe she doesn't belong in the "moderately-active" category. Referring back to the calorie chart, she finds the requirements for "sedentary" people: 10 calories per pound to maintain body weight. That is: $200 \times 10 = 2,000$. She is still aiming for a 3-pound loss every week, so once again she subtracts 1,500 calories from her basic caloric need. A total of 500 calories a day is practically a starvation diet, but like many fat people Nancy has a lot of willpower. After one week she loses all the weight she gained, except for half a pound. By the end of the second week of 500 calories a day she has lost that half pound, plus one more half pound. Three weeks on a diet—including two weeks of starvation dieting—and Nancy has lost eight ounces.

What Nancy has overlooked is the other element of

her body composition—Lean Body Mass. Although she weighs 200 pounds, she has only 90 pounds of Lean Body Mass (LBM); the rest is fat. LBM is muscle and bone. It is the actively metabolizing element of your body, and it requires a certain number of calories every day to stay in running order. The greater your LBM, the more calories you use (not store as fat, but *use*) every day. With only 90 pounds of LBM, sedentary Nancy needed only 900 calories per day to maintain her weight. To *lose* weight, of course, she would have to eat much less, and here the difficulty of low-calorie dieting emerges. Even if Nancy fasted for a week, she could not lose 3 pounds of fat simply by dieting. A 500-calorie starvation diet would eliminate 1 pound a week at most, and such a low-calorie diet would be tough to stick with for very long. After two or three weeks Nancy would probably give up, miserable and disgusted, and return to compulsive eating—and another 10 pounds of fat. Why not—her situation seems hopeless.

The fact is, Nancy—or anyone else—*can* succeed in losing weight and keeping it off. But not by dieting alone. You can only succeed by increasing your Lean Body Mass, which means improving your physical condition. Our combined diet and exercise program would work for Nancy in two ways. First of all, the test diet would reduce the amount of fat she's carrying around. Meanwhile, twenty-four minutes of daily exercise would soon increase Nancy's LBM to 120 pounds and her activity rating to "very active." This means she would require 20 calories per pound to maintain body weight (instead of 10 or 15), upping her basic caloric need to 2,400 calories, probably more than she is used to eating now. The point is, our patients do not just *lose fat*—any diet will eventually enable them to do that. They are *adding* calorie-burning Lean Body Mass. All of that additional muscle tissue means that the patient can safely eat up to 1,000 extra calories per day without gaining weight.

Although the change in your body's composition can be explained with facts and figures, the change in body chemistry you will undergo is more mysterious, though no less real. "Body chemistry" is a term that includes the thousands of chemical reactions that make our bodies work. A handful of these reactions have been isolated and analyzed; the rest have not. Many of these chemical reactions affect the absorption, utilization, assimilation, and excretion of food. Like the organic functions of your body, however, body chemistry can—and often *does*—operate imperfectly and reduce the efficiency with which your body handles food. Some of us are born with defective body chemistry. People who are short of an enzyme called lactase cannot drink milk without digestive problems. Juvenile diabetics who suffer from insulin deficiency cannot derive energy from sugar. But besides these congenital defects, I believe that many of us who were born perfectly healthy are suffering from *deteriorated* body chemistry. And the reason, I believe, is lack of physical fitness.

Medical science discovered long ago that sedentary people developed degenerative changes in their bodies. Muscles weaken; the heart, lungs, and blood vessels lose their elasticity; both energy and libido begin to dissipate. Now research is producing evidence that inactive people suffer not only physical but chemical deterioration.

In the past twenty years we've witnessed a dramatic increase in two diseases: adult-onset diabetes and hypoglycemia. These two diseases have many symptoms in common: both are associated with sugar metabolism and overproduction of insulin, and both are generally controlled with low-carbohydrate diets. Recently a prominent physician announced that he had successfully treated adult-onset diabetes by prescribing daily exercise, nothing more. He explained his success by saying that increased LBM gave the patient more tissue with which to burn off sugar. Impressed by his report, I tried the same program with eight of my patients who were hypoglycemics—and got the same results. Symptoms cleared up quickly, and within a few months all eight patients were able to go off whatever special diet had been prescribed. I attribute their improvement to exercise, which built up their LBM and thus normalized their body chemistry.

How does this research apply to you? Whether you are diabetic or not, physical fitness affects the efficiency with which your body handles food. In Week Three of the program's test diet you may discover that fruit makes you ravenous—so that eating a healthy-looking apple

23

quickly leads to cramming marshmallow cookies into your mouth. This means that, like me, you are probably a carbohydrate gainer: your sugar metabolism is defective, and you'll have to stay away from fruit and most other carbohydrates for a while. But once you achieve physical fitness, you should find, as I did, that your body chemistry has normalized. The natural sugar in fruit no longer unbalances your blood-sugar level, leaving you hungrier than you were before. Instead, your body is able to use carbohydrates as it would any other foodstuff, and you will be able to eat apples without bingeing afterward. This stabilization of chemistry will not take place overnight, but it *will happen*. The only catch is that you must continue to exercise every day of your life, twenty-four minutes a day. What we are talking about is a *temporary* test diet and a *permanent* exercise program.

If all this seems a bit fuzzy right now, just remember: dieting alone is a negative approach to weight loss; physical fitness is positive. The more LBM you have, the more calories you can accept into your system without converting them into stored fat.

Every fat person reading this book can succeed on the forty-nine-day program if he or she wants to. But each of you is starting out from a different place. Each of you is an individual, and although you are all overweight, you are overweight for different reasons and to different degrees. Since the most efficient health program is an individualized one, we will, as much as possible, be tailoring

24

both diet and exercise to your specific needs. But to do this, we have to find out more about why you—you *personally*—are fat. We need to know your habits, your tolerances, your strengths, your weaknesses. So, before we begin Week One's exercise and test diet, let's take some time to get better acquainted.

# Why Are *You* Fat?

This chapter is composed of five sets of questions. If you answer them truthfully, together we will find out what we need to know about you.

## OVEREATING

1. Do you feel you eat more than most of of your thin friends?
   (Much more, score 4; more, 3; the same, 2; somewhat less, 1; much less, 0.)                                        _____

2. Enter in the blank your total number of meals and snacks per day.                        _____

3.  a. How many slices of bread do you
        eat *per day*?                          _____

    b. How many potatoes? (Score 1 for
        each small white potato; 1 for each
        ½ cup mashed potatoes; 1 for each
        ¼ cup sweet potatoes or yams; 1 for
        each order of french fries.)            _____

    c. How many ounces of wine, whis-
        key, or other hard liquor do you
        drink? (Score 1 for every 4 ounces.)    _____

    d. How many scoops of ice cream do
        you eat? (Score 1 for every ½ cup.)     _____

    e. How much non-diet carbonated
        beverage do you drink? (Score 1
        for every 6 ounces.)                    _____

4.  Enter the approximate number of
    times a month you go on a binge and
    eat until you feel uncomfortably full.      _____

5.  Enter the number of times a week you
    finish a meal with dessert.                 _____

                                    TOTAL:      _____

If your score was: 12 or under: you are a light eater;
                   13 to 18: an average eater;
                   19 to 24: a heavy eater—the
                       amount of food you eat
                       is a definite factor in
                       your overweight;

25 or over: you overeat considerably and will have to pay strict attention to the size of your portions later in the diet program.

Most people who take this test at my clinic score as *light* eaters, although they are all anywhere from 25 to 150 pounds overweight. When I tell a patient he or she has scored low, I almost always hear an impassioned, sometimes bitter statement that goes something like this: "I've been telling my family for *years* that I don't eat much, but no one believes me. My husband insists I must be snacking all day, even though he can see I eat less than anyone else at dinner. Even our family doctor doesn't believe me!"

Studies have proven over and over again that most overweight people are *not* gluttons. But people who have never had a serious weight problem find this impossible to accept; they believe that double chins and gigantic thighs are unimpeachable evidence of overeating.

If you scored as a light or average eater, your problem may be that you are eating foods from a particular group that are wrong for your metabolism. If you are a heavy eater, you will learn new eating habits that will combat your tendency to overeat and, eventually, eliminate your need to do so.

## EATING HABITS

1. Do you eat alone? (If yes, score 1; if no, 0.) _____

2. Do you spend less than one half hour eating dinner? (Same scoring.) _____

3. Do you watch television while you eat? (Same scoring.) _____

4. Do you often eat standing up? (Same scoring.) _____

5. Do you often go to sleep within an hour after eating? (Same scoring.) _____

6. Do you feel compelled to eat everything on your plate? (Same scoring.) _____

TOTAL: _____

If your total is 2 to 4, then you have bad eating habits that probably caused you to score as a heavy eater on the Overeating quiz. If your score was 5 to 6, you either showed up as a heavy eater or you fibbed on several of the questions!

Many of our patients who overeat do so not because their appetites are monstrous but because they don't allow their bodies time to signal when they are full. Changing your eating habits will go a long way toward cutting down your food intake. Let me explain.

*Eating alone.* A solitary meal is usually an unwelcome and unhappy ceremony. It is a time when people feel most abandoned by the world. Many of us respond to this sense of loneliness by stuffing ourselves. For the busy executive who drags himself home late and sits down alone to warmed-over food, a full belly is security. To the wife who gives up waiting for her husband and eats alone, a heaping plate is solace. For the single person, a lonely meal can be the most awful part of the day.

Avoid the lonely meal. If you're married, don't eat alone in the kitchen. Skip the meal and make it up the next day together at breakfast. For the single person I advise finding someone to share meals with. We have long accepted the idea of car pools, so why not get together in eating pools?

*Eating fast.* This is a deadly habit. If you make up your mind to pace your meal so that it takes at least one half hour, you will find that you eat less. Food takes time to find its way into your bloodstream. As it does, it turns off your brain's hunger signals. If you eat too fast, you can consume many times what you need before your brain's satiety center gets the message that you don't need any more food. Many people have learned to recognize an uncomfortably stuffed feeling as the sign they have eaten enough. What they should become accustomed to is a *gradual* disappearance of hunger.

*Watching TV while you eat.* Tube-worship is an inadequate solution to the loneliness of eating by yourself and a terrible way to eat if you are with others. A meal must be a pleasant experience. You must slowly enjoy the good things before you. In one TV commercial the actors are asked what they had for dinner. No one remembers. Neither will you, if you're tuned in to the evening news. If you give time and attention to slowly savoring a meal, the memory of that meal will delay the onset of new hunger.

*Eating standing up.* If you won't take the time to pull up a chair, you certainly won't take the time to concentrate on your meal. If you catch yourself eating on the run, you can be sure you are on the way to overeating.

*Eating immediately before sleep.* Until we opened our clinic I never realized how many fat people doze right after dinner. Believe me, they shouldn't. Sleep sets the stage for perfect absorption of every calorie into your bloodstream—and for people who are trying to lose weight, that spells disaster. When you are asleep, neither the muscles nor the brain, which have top-priority claims on your blood supply, demands more than a minimum supply. As a result, blood vessels to the intestine open wide, and complete nutritional and caloric absorption takes place. What fat people should be trying for instead is greater *waste* of calories. Instead of allowing time for the bloodstream to absorb all those calories, they should be trying to empty their intestines as quickly as possible— and the way to do that is exercise. Instead of sleeping after dinner, take a walk. That, or any other mild activity, will deprive the intestine of full blood supply. Some calories will be absorbed, of course, but as much as 40 percent of the calories you consumed will pass quickly through your intestines and leave your body as waste.

*Cleaning your plate.* Test after test has proved that overweight people are compulsive about eating everything in sight. In one famous test, both fat and skinny people were asked to participate as subjects in a research experiment. What they didn't know was that the *real* experiment was taking place in the laboratory's waiting room. The assembled subjects were apologetically told that the start of the experiment had been delayed but that a lunch had been provided for them in the meantime. This ruse was used two days in a row, on two different groups of subjects. The first time, the researchers offered each subject one roast-beef sandwich and explained that there were more sandwiches in the refrigerator if anyone was still hungry. The fat subjects ate just one sandwich; the skinny subjects all went to the icebox and had another. The next day each subject was given a platter of three roast-beef sandwiches. This time the fat subjects ate every sandwich; the skinny subjects still ate only two.

This test and others like it show that overeaters are compulsive about eating everything on their plates. But the tests also indicate that while skinny people will eat until they are full, fat people eat until there is nothing more in sight—whether that involves one sandwich or three. Once you understand this odd fact about yourself,

32

you can turn it into an asset instead of a liability. When you sit down to a meal, put less food on your plate. If you've planned a roast for dinner, serve only as many slices as your family is likely to eat; leave the rest out of sight in the kitchen. As silly as it sounds, if there is not a lot of food right in front of you on the table, you will be content with much less. Sounds easy—and it is.

## ACTIVITY

1. How many times a week do you take an hour-long walk, bicycle half an hour, swim for fifteen minutes, or run for eight minutes *without* resting? (Score 7 for never exercising, 6 for once a week, and so on down to 0 if you exercise seven days a week.) _____

2. How many times a week do you nap in the afternoon (after eight hours' sleep the night before) or fall asleep while watching TV or reading after dinner? (Score 0 if never, on up to 7 for every evening.) _____

3. How many times a week do you pass up a social event because you feel too tired? _____

4. How many times a week do you work up a good sweat, in a game, or in some

33

aspect of your job, for example? (If you do it 7 times a week, enter 0; 6 times a week, enter 1; and if you never sweat because of any activity, enter 7. Do not count housework or sex, because they are usually not sustained for long enough periods of time.) _____

TOTAL: _____

If your score was: 7 or less: you have enough physical activity to sustain a strong body;

8 to 11: average;

11 to 15: you are not active.

Above 16: you are seriously inactive and this is probably having bad effects on both your weight and your health.

Most fat people are inactive. A team of scientists studying obesity in teen-age girls filmed some high school students as they played tennis and volleyball. The film showed that the researchers' obese subjects spent far more time standing motionless than did the players of average weight. No wonder. It's far more taxing to exercise when you are fat, yet inactivity and lack of exercise

34

contribute to keeping you that way. It's a vicious circle that must be broken if you are ever to be slim, strong, and, most important, healthy.

## HEREDITY

1.  When they were your age, were your grandfathers overweight? (For each grandfather up to 20 pounds overweight, add 10 points; up to 50 pounds, add 20 points; more than 50 pounds, add 30 points.)  _____

2.  Were your grandmothers overweight? (Use same scoring as you did for grandfathers.)  _____

3.  Were your parents overweight? (For each parent up to 20 pounds overweight, add 5 points; up to 50 pounds, add 10 points; more than 50 pounds, add 15 points.)  _____

TOTAL:  _____

If your score was:  0 to 25: heredity is not a primary cause of your weight problem;

26 to 40: heredity is a factor in your obesity;

Over 41 points: heredity is a serious obstacle for you, one that you will have to control and overcome through intelligent eating and exercise.

Statistics show that if one parent is overweight, about half the children will also be fat. If both parents are obese, chances are that two-thirds of their offspring will also be overweight.

Even if neither of your parents is fat, heredity may still be part of your problem, since obesity frequently skips one generation.

## HORMONES

First, some questions for women only:

1. Do you take birth-control pills? (If yes, score 20; if no, 0.)     ———

2. Do you take female hormones for postmenstrual symptoms? (If yes, score 20; if no, 0.)     ———

3. Do you have severe menstrual irregularity? (Score 7 for yes; 0 for no or not applicable.)     ———

4. Was your weight normal until you had your first baby? (Score 7 for yes, 0 for no or not applicable.)    _____
5. Was your weight normal until menopause? (Score 10 for yes; 0 for no or not applicable.)    _____
6. Are you afflicted with excess body hair? (Score 7 for yes, 0 for no.)    _____

TOTAL:    _____

If your score is over 27, you should discuss your weight problem with your gynecologist.

You may want to consider alternate methods of birth control. Going off the Pill will help you reduce, since you probably *gained* weight when you began taking it (most women gain at least five pounds). Also, certain feminizing hormones facilitate weight gain—in fact, they are similar to the hormones once used by ranchers to fatten up their cattle—and it's quite possible that your gynecologist can prescribe hormonal medication that offers the same beneficial effects without the unwelcome weight gain.

For men and women:
1. Was your weight normal until you reached puberty? (Score 7 for yes, 0 for no.)    _____

2. Do you take cortisone, or any similar medication such as Decadron, Medrol, or Aristocart? (Score 35 for yes, 0 for no.) _____

3. Do you take tranquilizers or antihistamines? (Score 7 for yes, 0 for no.) _____

4. Do you drink five or more cups of coffee or caffeine-containing diet drinks each day? (Score 7 if seven days a week, 6 for six days a week, etc.) _____

TOTAL: _____

If your score was: 14 or less: hormones are not a problem for you;

15 to 20: hormones are a minor problem, which won't seriously interfere with your ability to lose weight;

21 or over: hormones are a significant factor in your overweight.

I strongly suggest that you discuss your desire to lose weight with the doctor who prescribes your medication. You may be able to substitute sprays or inhalants for antihistamine pills. Cortisone medication increases appetite and aids water retention. If your condition is such that no other medicine can replace cortisone, weight loss *will* be more difficult for you, but not impossible.

I consider caffeine to be a very powerful drug. Caffeine, tranquilizers and antihistamines all affect production of insulin, which, in turn, affects blood-sugar level and appetite. A good step toward weight control is to cut down on caffeine. If you insist on coffee, postpone your first cup until the middle of the day. But what I really recommend is switching to caffeine-free products. You'll find you're not so tired in the middle of the day, and not so hungry at dinnertime or before bed.

If you take tranquilizers for emotional reasons, you and your doctor should consider that your weight problem is probably one significant reason for your anxiety and depression. If you discontinue them for the duration of this weight-loss program, you may feel so different about your life by the end of the program that such medication will no longer be necessary.

Now that we've discussed your eating and activity habits, as well as your background, we can begin to form an opinion about the causes of your weight problem.

Most of my patients are overweight because of a serious lack of exercise and because of heredity. Many doctors prefer to play down, or even deny, the importance of heredity, fearing it will make patients feel helpless or fatalistic. I disagree. Heredity *can* be overcome—*but not by dieting alone.* As I said before, overeating is usually the least significant factor.

If you are like our average patient, then, it is useless to attack only the most minor problem—the amount of food you eat—while ignoring the other, more important causes. You are not a glutton, so you will never lose weight permanently by dieting.

When the occasion was important enough to you (your approaching wedding? a short trip to a Caribbean island?) you found the willpower to starve yourself thin. Surely you can summon the determination you need now to follow a weight-loss plan that doesn't even ask you to do without your favorite foods!

Now is the time for you to decide whether or not you are ready to go ahead with a systematic program of diet, exercise, and education that will leave you with new habits, a new slim and healthy body, and a new life.

It's up to you.

# You Might Not Like It
# at First....

You will begin your exercise program by walking or riding a bicycle. That is all.

I realize that you probably will do everything in your power to avoid this physical activity. When I was fat, I did the same thing, quite successfully, too, until my heart warned me that I was killing myself.

You have a lot of company when it comes to avoiding physical activity. Statistics published by the President's Council on Physical Fitness show that only 6 percent of us flabby Americans ride bicycles, only 4 percent swim, and only 2 percent jog. Almost one-half of our adult population has never participated in a competitive sport, even while in school.

So it is understandable that, right now, you're very skeptical when I guarantee that after forty-nine days of regular physical activity you will feel better, look better, need less sleep, have more energy, and live a fuller life.

Even if you were not overweight, the idea of exercise would appear slightly abnormal to you. After all, people who exercise sweat. Their faces get red in public. They dash about, wearing shorts, running or bicycling when everyone around them is sitting in cars and on park benches, staring at the joggers as if they were visitors from another planet.

Perhaps you are secretly planning to skip the exercise portion of this plan and make up for it by depriving yourself of the piece of bread or the dessert the diet portion allows. THIS DOESN'T WORK! Even if you keep that promise to yourself and follow a stricter diet than I call for, *you can still gain weight if you do not increase your physical activity.*

Exercise is certainly a way to burn more calories immediately, but, more important, it will increase your lean body mass and alter your body's way of handling calories so that you will have more energy. This new energy is vital to successful weight loss because a person with energy is more active all day long. If you have a solid, muscular body, you will burn more calories just sitting still than a flabby, overweight person does. If eating carbohydrates—pizza, spaghetti, etc.—is disastrous for you now, you will suddenly find yourself able to eat these foods *without gaining weight* when you are in good physical condition.

Consider this example from my clinic.

Anne weighed 150 pounds, but 50 percent of her weight was fat, which requires very few calories to maintain itself. As a calorie burner, then, Anne was actually only a 75-pound woman.

As I explained on page 19, a sedentary person requires only 10 calories per pound per day to sustain body weight; a moderately active person needs 15 calories per pound per day; a very active person needs 20. Anne wasn't at all active, so she needed only 750 calories a day to maintain her weight. Her doctor put Anne on a 500-calorie starvation diet, but that gave her a daily deficit of only 250 calories.

Since 3,500 calories equal 1 pound, it was taking Anne *twelve days to lose 1 pound.* The largest actual fat loss she could hope for, after weakening herself and living in virtual deprivation for a prolonged time, was about 2½ pounds per month. One small candy bar, and Anne had eaten her day's supply of deficit calories. One big meal, and she would lose no weight at all that month!

Naturally, Anne felt terrible. She was grouchy and nervous most of the time. She was constantly hungry and thoroughly discouraged.

I could certainly sympathize with her. When I

weighed 220 pounds, I was 40 percent fat, meaning I needed only 1,320 calories per day to maintain my weight. On my 1,000-calorie diet, I had a mere 320 calories per day deficit, so a *month's* weight loss easily disappeared when I ate one—think of it! just *one*—pizza.

Besides, starvation diets do odd things to the human body. The body has survival instincts all its own; it doesn't want to be beautiful—it just wants to *be*. Thus, the moment you begin to starve yourself, your basal metabolism declines, so that your body requires even less energy to maintain its weight. If I needed 1,320 calories to maintain my body mass on a normal diet, I might need only 1,000 or 1,100 calories while starving myself—meaning I could be eating less and *still gain weight*.

But starvation is totally unnecessary. When Anne completed the forty-nine-day program, she weighed 120 pounds, and she still does. Now only 20 percent of her weight is fat. Her lean body mass has increased from 75 pounds to 96 pounds. She is now a very active person who requires 20 calories per pound per day to maintain her weight.

Anne now needs 1,920 calories per day to maintain her weight, as opposed to 750 calories when she started our program. She is 30 pounds lighter, yet she needs more than twice as many calories to keep up her present weight. Her heart is stronger, her muscle tone is healthy, she looks and feels younger.

More important, Anne is now living like a normal

44

person, eating almost everything she wants, while continuing to monitor her diet and remaining active. She has changed from a fat person, who eats little, is often hungry, and is usually tired, to a trim, fit person who has defeated her genes, enzymes, hormones, life-style, metabolism—all the causes of her obesity.

Dieting is immediately gratifying but is self-limiting in the long run. Increased physical activity is not immediately gratifying; in fact, it can be damned hard work. But, in the long run, it will become so satisfying that you will do it, not because it is prescribed but because you really want to. If you maintain your exercise plan for the first forty-nine days, I'm convinced that you will continue to exercise simply because you enjoy yourself. Exercise gives you positive feedback, it makes you feel good, whereas dieting offers only negative feedback, in the form of a fluctuating scale and endless hunger.

I'd like to anticipate your responses to my prescription of an exercise regimen. These are the classic ones I hear in my clinic every day.

*I don't have the time.* No one does. Ever. But when you actually begin regular physical activity sessions, you will soon see that you *must* have your riding, walking, or running time in order to have the energy you need to enjoy each day fully. You've always been able to find time for a nap when you were exhausted, haven't you? Once you feel increased energy through exercise, the prospect of returning to constant fatigue will be so appalling that your exercise period will become an absolute must.

*Exercise makes you hungrier, doesn't it?* No, no, no, no. Researchers have found that people who regularly avoid physical activity generally eat much more than their caloric requirements. But the kind of moderate exercise I prescribe, the same studies show, has just the opposite effect: it will decrease your appetite and make dieting easier.

*Isn't exercise dangerous? Can't it cause heart attacks?* What I am prescribing here is *moderate* physical activity, not doing a hundred push-ups or running until your legs collapse under you! You will begin exercising at a rate that is perfectly safe for *anyone*, no matter how out of condition, and progress *gradually*. Once you've completed the forty-nine-day plan, I suggest that you participate in sports and other physical activities. By then you will have learned how to monitor your own heart so that you will never overexert yourself.

If you are worried about your heart, keep in mind that what's *more* likely to provoke a coronary is *lack* of exercise.

*I keep promising to exercise and then I never do.* And you never will, unless you make exercise a convenient part of your day. Your physical activity can take as little as twenty-four minutes, depending on what you choose to do. But that time must be natural for you and must not interfere with your life-style to the point that the activity becomes a chore.

Think for a few minutes about how you can best fit your exercise regimen into your daily life. You'll have to decide what you can do without destroying your hairdo (probably the single most important obstacle to exercise among women!). Perhaps you'll switch to a hairdo that's easier to manage.

Many of my patients had similar doubts about finding time for exercise, but here are some examples of how they have incorporated physical activity into their lives:

—Frank, a stockbroker, parks his car two and a half miles from his office. This far from the center of the city, he always finds a space. He also saves twenty dollars a week in gas and parking fees. He walks as briskly as he can to work, taking slightly less than a half hour to get there, and the same amount of time to walk back after work. His first 30 pounds disappeared easily within forty-nine days, and his physical activity naturally became part of his daily schedule.

—Dave, a psychiatrist friend of mine, keeps his stationary bicycle in his office. Each of his patients has a fifty-minute session. Then, during the remaining ten minutes of each hour, Dave clears his mind by pedaling. Of course, Dave's patients may find it odd that he's slightly winded when their session with him begins, but Dave has certainly succeeded in making his exercise a convenient part of his day.

—Mike was so fat when he began the program that he felt too embarrassed to walk in his neighborhood. So he walked around inside his home. To lessen the tedium, Mike's children walked with him. He lost his first 40 pounds in two months and then felt confident enough to walk outdoors.

—Claude, our first 500-pounder, was a special problem for my clinic. The first time we asked him to walk one mile it took him twenty-seven minutes. He returned sweating and showed a pulse rate of 140, which was too fast for a man of his age and physical condition. We told Claude to slow down, even though he was already walking more slowly than anyone we had ever treated before. He bought special shoes for walking because he had never walked a mile before in his life. But he continued his walks.

Claude lost 75 pounds in the first two months. By then he was able to walk a mile in fifteen minutes. He now walks three miles during his lunch hour, thus burning calories and eliminating an opportunity to consume more. He continued with our program after the forty-nine days and to date has lost 140 pounds.

—When I began my own exercise program, I bought a stationary bicycle. Pedaling twenty-four minutes a day quickly became boring for me. Then I began watching television with my children in the morning. They ate breakfast and I cycled. That marvelously inventive program *Sesame Street* made the twenty-four minutes pass quickly and provided the subject for many fascinating conversations with my daughters.

*I won't walk when it's too cold or too hot outside. I can't ride a bicycle when it snows or rains. I'll exercise when I can, that's all.* Don't let the weather dictate to you. Use your imagination. People who want to swim can find indoor pools; people who bicycle can get a stationary cycle for wet days. People who enjoy walking or jogging can find an indoor track.

A stationary cycle, with speedometer and tension knob, is perfect for the beginning exerciser. You can pedal despite rain, sleet, snow, or gloom of night. And no one need see you until you feel ready to be seen.

Perhaps there is a sport or activity that interested you when you were younger. Would you consider finding a group of other adults who might play it with you?

I know I said "sport or activity," but for our purposes I must ask you to rule out such games as baseball or bowling. They are lots of fun, but neither provides the prolonged physical activity necessary to produce physical fitness. In baseball, most players spend most of the time either standing in the field or waiting to bat. They may have to run a short distance at top speed, but they never have to move for five or ten minutes without stopping. And bowlers are even worse. They spend most of the game seated, drinking beer and waiting to walk a few feet and roll a ball.

*Effective* physical activity means exercising without

interruption for enough time to force you to breathe in more oxygen than you normally do. How much time is "enough"? At the clinic we have found that twenty-four minutes of such activity has the best effects on the heart and circulatory system. Basketball, with its constant running, is a good cardiovascular activity (*but I do not advise playing basketball until after your first forty-nine days on this plan*).

Walking is the easiest, and stationary bicycling is best if you want to exercise at home.

Many of my patients buy dogs because they feel uncomfortable going for long walks alone. Not only is a dog a willing companion but he will serve as insurance against skipping your walk altogether. Princess *must* have her walk, and once you're out of the house the battle against your own laziness is half-won.

Whatever method you choose, I do not recommend —in fact, I strongly disapprove of—health clubs, where the beautiful machines do most of the work. Weight lifting and calisthenics (sit-ups, push-ups, chinning, toe-touches, etc.) might make you more limber and improve muscle tone, but because one tends to rest frequently between each set of exercises, these activities do not improve circulation or burn a significant amount of calories.

I have a friend who lives in Chicago's John Hancock Center whose idea of daily exercise is racing up the stairs to the hundredth floor. In *seventeen* minutes! Do *not* try this, or anything even half as strenuous. I want to stress that the kind of physical activity I am asking of you simply requires that you exert yourself continuously —but not furiously—twenty-four minutes a day for seven weeks. You should *not* push yourself. My friend is a doctor who knows the limits of his own body (if he *has* limits!). He is also in extraordinarily good physical condition. But you, for the moment, are not.

So much for the excuses. Remember, I have heard them all before, thought up by some of the best alibiers in the business. I don't buy it from them, and I won't from you. Never mind all the reasons you *can't* do your exercises. Start thinking of all the ways you *can*.

# Week One

## PHYSICAL ACTIVITY

This forty-nine-day beginning health program is about to attack your weight problem from two directions. This week you will begin your physical activity; by the end of the seventh week you probably will have worked up to doing twenty-four minutes a day. This week you will also begin a special seven-week diet. As I mentioned before, this diet will test your body's chemical reactions to the various food groups. It is also a low-calorie diet that will help you lose weight. The purpose of the two-pronged diet *and* exercise approach is this: at the same time that you are beginning to increase your Lean Body Mass, and thus your caloric needs, through exercise, you are also sharply decreasing your intake. This will result in the fairly dramatic weight loss most people need to keep up their spirits during a program of this kind. By the end of the program you will have reduced your weight considerably yet *increased* the number of calories you need to sustain it. You may even be able to abandon the diet, *as long as you continue to exercise* and keep one eye on what you eat.

Before beginning an exercise program, even one as moderate as this, you should visit your family doctor. Explain the program, discuss your medical history with him, and ask about your restrictions, if any. If you are over forty he may want to take an electrocardiogram, a painless test that monitors the electrical activity of your heart.

We are now at a critical point in this book.

You are anxious to start losing weight. You are excited about finding an alternative approach to starvation dieting.

But you know you probably can't get to see your doctor immediately, so you figure this is a good time to start the diet, but the exercise program can be shelved until the doctor comes back from vacation or until he has an appointment open.

*I don't want you to do that.*

I want you to begin your exercise program today.

Just as the Week One diet is specially designed just

to get you started, your first week of physical activity is a mild, perfectly safe warm-up *that can be performed by anyone who can walk.*

Call your doctor today and make an appointment. As soon as you hang up, go out and take your first half-hour walk. You can't work diligently at the diet portion of this plan and ignore the exercise; you must start both at the same time.

Many of my patients schedule their walk just before dinner because physical activity decreases appetite. A glass or two of water after your walk will cut your appetite even more. This will be a big help, because dinner is usually the largest meal of the day.

During your walk, don't stop at the dry cleaners or the grocery, or for a chat with your neighbor. Without overtaxing yourself, walk briskly and purposefully. I say that you shouldn't stop during your walk, but I do want you to pause and check your heart rate at least twice in the half hour. It only takes fifteen seconds, so you won't really be interrupting your exercise.

Below is a list of what are called "training rates"— that is, you may safely speed your heartbeat up to these limits during exercise periods. You will benefit most from your exercise if the exertion *does* cause your heart to reach the limits prescribed for your age. *Memorize the rate that applies to you.* During your exercise you will be checking your pulse regularly to make sure you have reached these limits without exceeding them.

| AGE | HEARTBEATS PER MINUTE |
|---|---|
| 20–24 | 150–165 |
| 25–29 | 145–160 |
| 30–34 | 140–155 |
| 35–39 | 135–150 |
| 40–44 | 130–145 |
| 45–49 | 125–140 |
| 50–54 | 122–135 |
| 55–59 | 117–130 |
| 60–64 | 110–125 |
| over 65 | 105–120 |

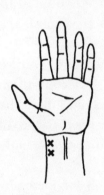

To take your pulse, grasp either of your wrists on the palm side with the first and second fingers of the other hand. On the thumb side of the wrist you will feel a bone. If you move about a quarter of an inch down, toward your little finger, you will feel your pulse. If you move too far down, you will feel a cordlike tendon in the middle of your wrist. Between the tendon and the bone, you should find your pulse. Count the beats for fifteen seconds and multiply by four.

If you have exceeded your limit, slow down, but do not stop completely. Take it easy and wait for your pulse rate to decrease to safe limits. If at any time you feel dizziness, nausea, or lightheadedness, stop and take your pulse.

Walk for thirty-five minutes on the second day and forty minutes on the third day.

When you can walk for forty minutes without stopping—being careful to stay within the correct training limits—then gradually increase your speed until you can cover two miles in that forty minutes. You will probably be able to do this within the first week, but if you can't, don't be discouraged. Take as long as you need, but work at it. *Two miles in forty minutes is your first physical activity goal.*

If you choose to bicycle outdoors, ride two miles the first day, taking as long as you need to accomplish that distance.

Each day increase your cycling speed until you can do two miles in less than ten minutes. (Of course, you can ride longer or go farther, but you should isolate that ten-minute, two-mile ride as your physical activity goal.

If you prefer a stationary cycle, ride at twelve miles per hour, and try to go for two miles.

Most stationary bicycles have a knob for increasing or decreasing resistance to pedaling. As you pedal, your legs may start to get tired. When this happens, relax the tension until you can pedal comfortably again. After a few minutes, tighten the tension gradually. If your legs begin to ache, ease off the tension. The tension should be set so that it is a little less than the amount necessary to make your legs ache.

Try to hold your speed at twelve miles per hour. But if

56

you feel that your heart is beating too fast, take your pulse. If you have exceeded your training limit, slow down and allow your heart rate to return to the proper range. After six days, you will probably be able to pedal the complete two-mile distance at twelves miles per hour without exceeding the limits set for your heart.

On the seventh day of Week One you will test yourself to see if you're ready to go on to the Week Two exercise program. Week One's goals shouldn't be too difficult for you, and most of my patients are ready for Week Two after the first six days of exercise. I'll discuss this test in the Week Two chapter (pages 83–117).

Meanwhile, you have a goal to accomplish as quickly as possible: if you are walking, you want to walk two miles in forty minutes; if you're cycling, outdoors or in, you want to pedal two miles in ten minutes.

You are at the beginning of a long road back to physical fitness. Do the exercises patiently and persistently. Don't try to accomplish everything today. Don't be discouraged if you don't feel in top physical shape within a few days. Your immediate satisfaction will be coming from a relatively large weight loss on the Week One diet. The benefits of the conditioning program won't begin to show themselves until around the fourth week of the plan but, as I've mentioned before, those benefits are enormous.

The exercise you are doing will burn only about 75 calories. This is not a significant amount, but burning calories is not the purpose of your exercise. What we are really aiming for is an increase in Lean Body Mass, the muscular, solid portion of your body that burns calories quite actively. Remember: as LBM increases, so does the number of calories you can eat without gaining weight.

As you become physically fit, you will also feel more energetic. Your afternoon and after-dinner naps will cease, and you'll find yourself more and more active during the day. The resulting increase in your daily activities will burn more calories per day than you did before, and this, too, will up the number of calories you can eat without gaining.

As you approach physical fitness, the wonderful gift of energy you will feel should confirm for you all that I've said.

## THE STARTER DIET

Now that you've been briefed on your physical-activity goal for Week One, we can turn to our second plan of attack: your diet.

The Week One Starter Diet is *not* part of the test diet. It is a low-calorie diet designed to take weight off quickly and provide psychological momentum. It is not an adequate long-term diet. You *must* go on to Week Two after seven days on Week One.

You may be impressed with your weight loss in the first week, and this loss may lure you into remaining on

Week One so that you can continue to lose quickly. *This will not happen.* What *will* happen is that the Week One diet will soon leave you too tired to continue exercising; once that happens, your weight loss will hit a plateau, and you will become disgusted and sack the whole project.

So I ask you to trust me, trust this plan, and abandon Week One at the end of Week One!

I conduct Week One in two ways, depending on the needs of my patients. To some I simply offer a list of the foods that are allowable. Others, however, feel they need more guidance in order to stick with the plan in this first, crucial week. For those patients I have prepared a complete seven-day menu, including recipes, which are listed in the back of this book.

I don't believe in regimenting what people eat, because it is impossible to find two people with the same tastes in food. So use the menu I've developed if you like, and depart from it where you need to. I say depart from the *menu*, mind you, but *not* from the food list.

## THE WEEK ONE DIET

You may have only two meals each day.

During Week One, use *no* butter, margarine, oil, shortening, or sugar. (Don't worry—these foods will all be restored to your diet in Week Five, except sugar, which will reappear in Week Seven.)

GROUP ONE: FRUIT.    *Choose 1 each day:*

½ grapefruit
1 apple
1 orange
½ cup fresh strawberries

GROUP TWO: MEAT.    *Choose 2 each day:*

1 8-ounce chicken breast
1 6-ounce steak, trimmed of fat
1 16-ounce piece of fish
1 egg
1¼ cups cottage cheese

GROUP THREE: VEGETABLES.    *Choose 2 each day:*

| | | | |
|---|---|---|---|
| Asparagus | Cauliflower | Escarole | Radish |
| Beans, string | Celery | Lettuce | Sauerkraut |
| Broccoli | Chicory | Mushrooms | Spinach |
| Brussels sprouts | Cucumbers | Okra | Squash, summer |
| Cabbage | Eggplant | Pepper, green | Tomatoes |
| | | | Watercress |

GROUP FOUR: BREAD.    *Choose 1 each day:*

1 breadstick
1 piece Melba toast

You may use the following in unlimited amounts throughout the forty-nine-day plan:

Any herb or spice, lemon juice, vinegar, artificial sweeteners, dietetic sodas (with *no* sugar), coffee, tea, Sanka, water, bouillon.

You might enjoy lemonade made from the juice of 1

lemon combined with one cup of water and sweetened artificially.

## THE WEEK ONE MENU

I believe that eating—especially on a diet—should be a pleasant experience. You should prepare your table carefully and eat only when you are seated. Your meals should look inviting. There's a very great difference, psychologically, between eating cottage cheese straight from the plastic container and arranging it with fresh fruit on a china plate. You'll see.

Sit down, unfold your napkin, and *eat slowly*. Spend at least twenty minutes at each meal. In your brain are both a hunger center and a satiation center. Give your satiation center time to register everything you are eating, and you will feel fuller at the end of your meal.

Remember the Eating Habits quiz? Turn off the TV and turn on to your food.

*(See the lettered recipes, which follow on pages 229-240.)*

| | | | |
|---|---|---|---|
| DAY ONE | Meal 1 | A | Egg with Mushroom Filling |
| | | B | ½ Grapefruit, Sectioned Beverage |
| | Meal 2 | C | Ruffled Salad |
| | | D | Chicken Imperial |
| | | E | Broccoli Italienne |
| DAY TWO | Meal 1 | F | Eve Salad Breadstick |

|  |  |  |  |
|---|---|---|---|
|  | Meal 2 | G | Magic Mushroom Salad |
|  |  | H | Steak Pacifica |
|  |  | I | Lemon Green Beans |
| DAY THREE | Meal 1 | J | Riviera Salad |
|  |  | K | Baked Perch Italiano |
|  |  |  | Melba toast |
|  | Meal 2 | L | Broiled Herb Chicken |
|  |  | M | Swedish Spinach |
|  |  |  | Fresh Orange Segments |
| DAY FOUR | Meal 1 | N | Tomato à la Russe |
|  |  |  | Melba Toast |
|  | Meal 2 | O | Beef Stroganoff |
|  |  | P | Stuffed Mushrooms |
|  |  |  | Orange |
| DAY FIVE | Meal 1 | Q | Sunshine Salad |
|  |  | R | Chicken Rosemary |
|  | Meal 2 | K | Baked Perch Italiano |
|  |  |  | Asparagus |
|  |  |  | Breadstick |
| DAY SIX | Meal 1 | S | Snowdrift Salad |
|  |  | T | Egg with Tomato |
|  | Meal 2 | U | Hickory Steak |
|  |  | V | Tomato Provençale |
|  |  |  | Apple |
| DAY SEVEN | Meal 1 | W | Egg with Zucchini |
|  |  | X | Emerald Salad |
|  | Meal 2 | Y | Oriental Chicken Salad |

## THE END OF WEEK ONE

### Are You Getting Enough to Eat?

The Week One Diet may not seem like much to eat when you read over the list, but many patients find it leaves them comfortably full. I'm not surprised by this reaction to the diet, because I know that fat people are accustomed to starving themselves.

This week's diet averages only 500 calories a day. If you're getting enough to eat this week, that means you have a very low caloric requirement; you can see how very little food you require to maintain your fat. Dieting alone is never going to work for you. You must exercise to increase the number of calories you burn if you are ever going to lose weight and keep it off.

If, on the other hand, you aren't satisfied by Week One's meals, eat more from the vegetable A group listed on page 99. Those vegetables have minimal calories but provide bulk to fill you up.

Eating these vegetables in quantity may seem to slow your weight loss, because they are largely water by weight. But although your scale may not be registering weight loss, this water retention will *not* interfere with the amount of fat you are taking off your body this week. As long as you are exercising and sticking to the diet, you *are* burning fat, regardless of what your scale shows.

If you're hungry during Week One, don't be discouraged. In the next few weeks, you'll be getting more and more filling foods, I promise.

## How Much Weight Have You Lost?

### *3 Pounds or Less*

Everyone who followed the diet exactly will have lost 3½ to 5½ pounds of fat, even if the scale doesn't show it. As I've mentioned, your body tries to protect its weight and may react to a low-calorie diet by lowering your calorie-burning rate (metabolic rate), or by retaining water. At some point in the next forty-nine days, your body *will* give up the water and your scale will indicate a marked loss at that time.

If you would feel better, however, seeing your weight decrease on your bathroom scale, you can help rid your body of excess fluid by drinking more non-salty liquids—water, decaffeinated coffee, tea. All this liquid will push your body to its saturation point, when it will be able to retain no more water. At that point you will begin eliminating water in your urine and your true weight loss will show up on the scale.

If you are working toward water loss, *avoid* salt and salt-containing liquids (like diet drinks, whose salt content is substantial). Because of the chemical attraction between salt and water, salt is an important factor in water retention.

Try to drink eight to twelve cups of non-salty fluids

per day. If you really find this impossible (if your desk isn't near the rest room, you'll do a lot of walking), just hang on and be confident; you *are* burning fat, and it will show soon.

## 3½ to 5½ Pounds

Your scale has been honest; you haven't held back water that might disguise your loss. If you feel that this isn't much to lose, think about it: at the end of the forty-nine days, you will have lost 25 to 35 pounds, and you'll be eating more and more food in each of the remaining weeks!

## Over 5½ Pounds

You're thrilled and overjoyed. Some of my patients have lost as much as 20 pounds in the first week, and I always try to bring them down to earth right away. You are not going to continue to lose at this rate through the remaining weeks of the plan. No one can lose more than 5½ pounds of actual fat in one week; what you have lost in the first week is a lot of water. This means that if you lost 10 pounds this week, chances are you won't register any loss at all next week, because your water loss is already over. You may even *gain* a pound after doing everything right. Just remember that you haven't stopped burning fat, you've just stopped losing water. Don't let your scale overly affect your spirits.

Try to concentrate on your weight-loss goal at the end of the forty-nine days.

## If Your Weight Goal Is Less Than 30 Pounds

You probably know very well what your perfect weight is—in fact, you've probably been there a few times in the last five years. Continue to strive for that goal. But you should set a clothing-size goal for yourself, too. You might be surprised to find that you'll reach your desired size long before your desired weight.

Replacing fat with Lean Body Mass will result in a more compact and shapely you, even if your weight still hasn't come down as far as you would like. When you get right down to it, the way you *look* is what really counts. Let's say you were overweight but had a figure like Raquel Welch's. Would you really care what the scale said?

I've had patients who worked down to the smallest clothing sizes they'd ever worn but still felt defeated because the scale did not show them what they wanted to see. Your waistline can tell you more about your progress than your scale.

## If Your Weight Goal Is More Than 30 Pounds

You are going to take a lot of weight off quickly, but at the end of forty-nine days you will still have work to do.

You should have two goals: first, to complete the forty-nine-day plan; and second, to reach your desired weight. In forty-nine days, you should lose 30 pounds.

Determine your second goal as follows:

Allow 105 pounds for the first five feet of your height and 6 pounds for each inch over five feet. If you are five feet six inches tall, you should weigh 105 pounds for the first five feet, plus 6 pounds for each of the additional six inches, or 141 pounds.

These figures are a rough rule of thumb. Many of you will still feel fat when you have reached your goal. Others of you will feel that you have lost enough long before you reach that weight. Your correct weight can only be determined by certain precise scientific techniques. Short of that, the best way to determine a goal is to find a weight at which you are satisfied with the way you look.

But let's concentrate on getting those first 30 pounds off. Toward the end of this book we will talk about how to continue losing weight after the forty-nine days are over.

# The Basics
# of Exchange Dieting

Which will cause you to gain more weight: a piece of bread with two pats of butter; a half cup of ice cream; or an average-size chocolate bar?

If you said that they all contain the same number of calories and the same amount of protein, carbohydrates, and fat, then you already know something about exchange dieting, one of the most flexible diets ever devised.

The dieters' bible can be summarized in a single commandment: *Know foods.* Know how many calories, proteins, carbohydrates, and fats compose the foods you normally eat.

There are really only two ways to supply yourself with this information. An expert nutritionist could fill in mimeographed sheets detailing exactly what you could eat, when, and in what amounts. The inconvenience and expense to the patient aside, the expert would have to devote a good part of his life to endlessly filling out the information sheets, or the patient would soon be eating the same monotonous meals each day.

A better approach is to teach the *dieter* a lot about food, as quickly and efficiently as possible, so that he or she can rapidly calculate the calories and the proteins, carbohydrates, and fats in every food.

This is what exchange dieting will teach you. You will start looking upon food in terms of "exchanges" that will automatically count calories, fats, carbohydrates, and proteins. You will learn that a six-ounce Coca-Cola equals one slice of bread and that a chocolate milk shake equals five slices of bread and butter.

And you'll begin switching easily to satisfying foods that are less costly in terms of calories, thus losing weight with really little effort at all.

The biggest advantage of the exchange-diet method is that, after a surprisingly short learning period, it is so simple. This is a boon to veteran dieters who are tired of desperately leafing through the calorie- or carbohydrate-counting tables they've grown accustomed to carrying about in their handbags or hip pockets.

To teach you the basics of exchange dieting as quickly

as possible, I will ask you to do something you probably haven't done since school (something besides exercising, that is). I will ask you to take a test to make sure that you have understood what you have read.

If you follow the directions, you will become actively involved in the material and will retain the information much longer than if you read it presented in the ordinary manner. This is something I've found to be true again and again in my clinic. Taking the time to write down answers to questions ensures that you really are absorbing what you are reading.

Some questions are very easy and you may be tempted not to answer them. Try not to give in. Even the most difficult theories are based on simple principles, and while I may not be quizzing you on highly technical matter, there *are* some complexities to exchange dieting. These will be easier for you if you have a thorough understanding of the basics and have proven that understanding to yourself by answering all the questions.

The correct answers are printed to the left of the questions; cover the answer column with a piece of paper or your hand. Write your response to each question in the space provided, or circle the appropriate word or term. Then move the paper or lift your hand to reveal the correct answer on the left.

If you make a mistake, cross out your answer and write the correct answer above it. Take as much time as you like, but try not to look at the printed answer before you have given your own response.

What you are about to learn here will eventually enable you to design a diet for yourself, one suited to your own individual tastes and needs. I have said before that I don't believe it's possible to remain on a regimented diet indefinitely. An understanding of exchange dieting will be your ticket to freedom from all the diets that have deprived you of the foods you will never stop loving.

This will be your very last diet book.

|  |  |
|---|---|
| calories | 1. Calories are units that measure *energy*. All foods contain cal____. Therefore all foods provide the body with *energy*. |
| energy, calories | 2. En____ is measured in units called ca____. |
| more, energy | 3. All foods contain a certain number of calories. Since the number of calories in a food measures how much energy that food supplies to the body, it follows that the (*fewer/ more*) calories a food contains, the more e____ it supplies to the body. |
| calories | 4. The more cal____ a food con- |

energy

tains, the more  e_____  it will supply to the body.

more

5. Since it takes (*fewer/more*) calories to enable the body to do more
work, a professional athlete would

more

require a diet containing (*more/
fewer*) calories than a typical office
worker would, because an athlete
uses more energy than an office
worker.

energy

6. In other words, the more  e_____
a person expends during the course

calories

of a day's activity, the more  cal_____
he requires in his diet.

7. Beth Goddard is a draftswoman.
For many hours a day, she sits at a
drawing board. After work, she enjoys going to movies, reading, and

less

watching TV. She uses (*more/less*)
energy than a professional athlete
and therefore requires a diet that is

lower

(*lower/higher*) in calories than an
athlete's diet.

8. Mr. Stockton is a bricklayer who
enjoys tennis, swimming, and horse-
back riding. Mr. Stockton uses

more

more

(*more/less*) energy than a typical office worker and therefore requires a diet containing (*more/fewer*) calories than an office worker's diet.

calories

energy

9. In most people, the number of cal_____ a person consumes in his daily food intake almost exactly equals the number of calories his body needs to produce e_____ to get through the day's activities. When a person has achieved this calorie-energy balance, his weight remains *stable* over a long period of time.

stable

calories

energy

10. A st_____ body weight is a good indication that your body is using all the cal_____ contained in your daily intake of food as e_____.

stable

11. Jill Hansen has weighed 117 pounds for six years. Her body weight can therefore be considered st_____.

73

12. When a person has had the same body weight for a long period of time, it usually means that the

calories

number of cal_____ contained in his daily intake of food closely approximates the number of calories

energy

his body needs to use as e_____ to get through the day's activities.

13. So, if a person used all the

calories
energy
stable

cal_____ contained in his daily intake of food as e_____ , his body weight would be st_____ .

14. If a person consumes more

calories

cal_____ than are required for the day's activity, he will store the re-

calories

maining cal_____ in the form of fat.

15. When enough calories are not supplied in the diet for the day's activity, the calories will be drawn

fat

from the body's supply of f_____ . If body fat is used to supply suffi-

energy

cient calories as e_____ for the day's activity, a person will lose weight. If calories are stored as fat

f _____ , because a person needs fewer calories for the day's activity than he eats, the person will become

heavier

(*heavier/lighter*).

16. If a stable body weight can only be maintained when the number of calories used by the body to produce energy is roughly equal to the number of calories contained in a person's daily diet, what would you predict about the body weight of a person who doubled his caloric intake and decreased his level of activity?

a. He would lose weight.

b. He would
gain weight.

b. He would gain weight.

c. His body weight would remain stable.

17. Dave Alpert is promoted from an outdoor job that required vigorous physical activity to a managerial position that requires sitting at a desk most of the day. Although his level of activity has decreased considerably, he still consumes the same number of calories in his daily

increase

diet. If he continues to do so, his body weight will probably (*decrease/increase*).

18. It is possible, then, to depart from your ideal weight in a number of ways. If you increase your caloric intake by eating (*more/less*) food and do not also increase your level of activity, you will probably (*gain/lose*) weight.

more

gain

19. If you eat less food and thereby (*increase/decrease*) the number of calories you consume while at the same time you expend more energy by increasing your level of activity, you will probably (*lose/gain*) weight.

decrease

lose

20. The calories contained in any food are supplied by three basic foodstuffs: *fats, carbohydrates, and proteins.* That is, the number of calories contained in any food depends upon the number and the kind of the three basic f_____ that make up the food.

foodstuffs

21. All foods contain varying amounts and kinds of the three basic

foodstuffs

f⎯⎯⎯. It is the relative quantity of these three basic elements that is responsible for the number of

calories

cal⎯⎯⎯ contained in any food.

22. The caloric content of any food is determined by the amount and kind of the three basic foodstuffs (fats, carbohydrates and proteins) contained in that food. All foods contain one or more of these three basic foodstuffs. Bread, for example, contains carbohydrates and proteins

fats

but does not contain f⎯⎯⎯.

23. Oranges contain only one of the basic foodstuffs. They do not contain fats or proteins. Therefore

carbohydrates

oranges contain only ca⎯⎯⎯.

24. Pears, and most other fruits, are similar to oranges in that they do

fats

not contain f⎯⎯⎯ or proteins but

carbohydrates

do contain ca⎯⎯⎯.

25. Eggs contain two of the basic foodstuffs but do not contain any

fats

proteins

carbohydrates. Eggs contain f ____

and pr_____ .

carbohydrates,

fats, proteins

26. Cottage cheese and eggs are similar in that they contain the same two basic foodstuffs and lack the same basic foodstuff. Cottage cheese and eggs do not contain any ca_____ , but do contain f_____ and pr_____ .

56

27. When nutritionists refer to the amount of fats, carbohydrates, and proteins in any food, they use a unit of weight called the gram. In 1 ounce there are 28 grams. In 2 ounces there are _____ grams.

weight

28. Grams are a unit of w_____ , just like pounds or ounces, but they are smaller.

28

29. One ounce contains _____ grams while ½ ounce contains 14 grams.

30. The abbreviation for gram is gm. If we were to use this short-ened form to write the number of grams in an ounce, we would write

gm.                      28 _____ .

31. How many grams in 1 ounce? Circle one:

28                12      28      36      0

32. So far we have learned two units of measure for food. One is called the gram, which is a measure

weight          of w _____ .

33. The other unit of measure we

calorie        have learned is the cal _____ ,

energy         which measures e _____ .

34. The unit of measure of energy,

calorie        which is called the cal _____ , and the unit of measure of weight,

gram           which is called the g _____ , are re- lated. Each gram of the same food- stuff supplies a fixed amount of energy. For example, 1 gram of pro- tein yields four calories.

four            35. Protein, then, contains fo _____ calories to the gram. Since there are 28 grams in an ounce, how many calories would there be in 1 ounce

$28 \times 4 = 112$    of protein? _____ .

36. Carbohydrates and proteins contain the same number of calories per gram. Both carbohydrates and proteins contain fo_____ calories to the gram.

four

37. Circle the number of calories per gram contained in both carbohydrates and proteins:

4

4    6    3    5

$7 \times 4 = 28$
$2 \times 4 = \phantom{0}8$
$\overline{\phantom{00}36}$

38. How many calories are in ½ cup of cooked carrots, which contains 7 gm. carbohydrates and 2 gm. proteins?

39. Carbohydrates and proteins contain fo_____ calories to the gram, while the remaining basic foodstuff, f_____, contains nine calories to the gram.

four

fat

40. Since 1 gram of fat contains n_____ calories, how many calories are in 9 grams of fat? _____

nine
$9 \times 9 = 81$

41. Match the foodstuff listed below with the correct number of

calories contained in 1 gram of that foodstuff:

c. 9

b. 4

b. 4

fats _____        a. 6

proteins _____        b. 4

carbohydrates _____        c. 9

d. 12

$12 \times 4 = 48$

$8 \times 4 = 32$

$10 \times 9 = 90$

$\overline{170}$

42. How many calories are in 1 cup of milk, which contains 12 gm. carbohydrates, 8 gm. proteins, and 10 gm. fat? _____.

These basics of exchange dieting are a tool you will be using, not only for the rest of the forty-nine days, but as long as you continue to diet. Once you are sure you've mastered them, you are ready to begin the dieting experiment that starts right now, in Week Two.

# Week Two

## WEEK TWO DIET

During Week One you followed a simple low-calorie diet designed to start you off with an encouraging weight loss. In Week Two, however, you will begin the "test diet," which, besides helping you lose *now*, will teach you what you need to know about yourself in order to *keep* weight off until you reach physical fitness.

The six-week test diet is organized around the seven basic food groups. As I mentioned earlier, all foods are grouped by the type and amount of proteins, carbohydrates, and fats they contain. The groups are: *meat, vegetables A and B, fruit, fat, milk,* and *bread.* Meat contains protetin and fat; fruit is entirely carbohydrate. Vegetables have moderate amounts of carbohydrate and some protein; Vegetable B's are higher in carbohydrates. Milk contains all three foodstuffs—fat, protein, and carbohydrate, which is why grammar school teachers call it the perfect food. Bread is largely carbohydrate, with a small amount of protein. (A few vegetables that are very high in carbohydrate—like corn and potatoes—are part of the bread group.) And fat, of course, is nothing but fat.

So that you can learn about each of these groups, we will add one to the diet each week. In this way, you will become aware of the effects of each type of food on your system.

In the Week Two diet (actually the first week of testing your responses to the food groups) you will eat foods only from the meat and vegetable A groups. You will be eating exclusively from these two groups for the next seven days.

That doesn't mean that your diet will be restricted to meat and vegetables, however. Cheese, eggs, fish, and poultry are also part of the meat group, so there should be enough diversity to please everyone. For the next forty-two days, eat only the foods *listed* for the various groups. In the chapter titled "Some Fancy Exchange Dieting" you will learn how exchange dieting enables you to eat anything you like. But for now, eat only what is on the list for each group.

We're going to start with a learning program on meat exchanges. This is the same format you used to learn about the basics of exchange dieting, so cover the answers in the column on the left and begin.

1. Each of the foods in the meat group has the same amount of fats, proteins, and calories. This means that you can eat any food in the meat group in place of any other food in the group. The foods on the meat-group list are called meat exchanges. Write "meat exchanges" in the space provided:

exchanges

2. Foods in the meat group are called meat ex_____ because any food on the list can be eaten in place of any other food on the list, provided it is eaten in proportionate quantity.

exchange

3. One egg and 1 ounce of *cooked* beef are both equal to one meat ex_____ . This means that if you wanted, you could eat an egg instead of an ounce of cooked beef.

**84**

4. The distinction between cooked beef and uncooked beef is important because meats shrink when they are cooked. This shrinkage usually amounts to about 25 percent. Figuring this 25 percent shrinkage, how much would 4 ounces of beef weigh after it was cooked? Circle one:

¼ of 4 = 1

4 − 1 = 3

3 ounces

|  |  |
|---|---|
| 2 ounces | 4 ounces |
| 3 ounces | 5 ounces |

25

3

5. Meat shrinks about _____ percent when it is cooked. This means that 4 ounces of beef (¼ pound) would weigh about _____ ounces after it is cooked. (You should have a small kitchen scale and always weigh your meat after it has been cooked. If you weigh your food before you cook it, you'll be cheating yourself out of about 25 percent of the food you are entitled to. Most restaurants feature what they call a "quarter-pound [4-ounce] hamburger." Remember that this is the weight of the meat before it is cooked, and that hamburgers in most restaurants are equal to *three*

85

meat exchanges, since 1 ounce of cooked meat equals one meat exchange.

6. In the previous section you learned that each gram of protein contains 4 calories and each gram of fat contains 9 calories. One meat exchange contains 7 grams of protein and 5 grams of fat. Using this information, how many calories are contained in one meat exchange? Enter your answer in this space: _____ calories in one meat exchange.

$$7 \times 4 = 28$$
$$5 \times 9 = 45$$
$$\overline{\phantom{0}73}$$

7. Each meat exchange contains 7 grams of protein. Thus five meat exchanges would contain _____ grams of protein.

35

8. Circle the number of grams of protein contained in one meat exchange:

7

6      3      7      1

9. Each meat exchange contains 5 grams of fat. Five meat exchanges,

25

then, would contain _____grams of fat.

10. Circle the number of grams of fat contained in one meat exchange:

5

4    6    5    1

five, seven,
calories

11. Each meat exchange contains fi _____ grams of fat, se _____ grams of protein, and 73 cal _____ .

exchange

12. One egg and 1 ounce of beef both contain 7 grams of protein and 5 grams of fat. This is the same number of fats and proteins as are contained in one meat ex _____ .
Since an egg and an ounce of beef contain identical amounts of fats and proteins, it follows that they also contain equal amounts of

calories

cal _____ , because the caloric content of food is dictated by the fats, carbohydrates, and proteins it contains.

13. An egg and an ounce of beef are both equal to one meat ex-

fats,                change. This means that they both
contain equal amounts of f _____ ,
proteins, calories    p _____ , and cal _____ .

You can see now that "meat exchange" is a very handy term, because it describes not only the number of calories in a food, but also the amount and kind of foodstuffs contained in that food.

Below you will find a chart of the meat exchange equivalents. All the allowable foods are listed in amounts equal to one meat exchange. You will need this information for the meat exchanges on your Week Two diet. The next set of questions will be based on the chart, so you will have to refer back to it in formulating your answers.

### MEAT EXCHANGE EQUIVALENTS
*Each Item Equals One Meat Exchange*

| | |
|---|---|
| Any meat or poultry (medium-fat) | 1 ounce |
| Cold cuts (4½″ x ⅛″) | 1 slice |
| Frankfurter (8–9 per pound) | 1 |
| Egg | 1 |
| Any fresh fish | 2 ounces |
| Canned fish | ¼ cup |
| Shellfish (shrimp, clams, oysters, etc.) | 5 small |
| Any cheese ° | 1 ounce |
| Cottage cheese | ¼ cup |

° *Except cream cheese, which contains much more fat than the foods in the meat group. Cream cheese will be added later, in the fat group.*

1.  Kathy Russo has planned a diet that allows her to eat 7 meat exchanges a day. Following is a list of the foods from the meat list that she plans to eat in one day. In the spaces provided, list how many exchanges each food is worth, referring back to the Meat Exchange Equivalents list if necessary:

2 ounces of beef:

2 _____exchanges

¼ cup cottage cheese:

1 _____exchanges

6 ounces mackerel:

3 _____exchanges

1 ounce Cheddar cheese:

1 _____exchanges

2.  How many meat exchanges are in a salad comprised of 10 small shrimp, ¼ cup cottage cheese, and 1 egg? Circle one (refer back to the Meat Exchange Equivalent list if necessary):

4        5     4     3     6

3.  Suppose you want to use only 2 meat exchanges at your next meal

and you may choose from the three following dishes. Which one would you choose in order not to violate your self-imposed limitation? Underline one:

a. A 3-egg omelette
b. 3 ounces of roast chicken

c. 4 ounces
whitefish

c. 4 ounces of whitefish

4. Bob Edwards is a busy salesman who must attend buffet lunches occasionally in the course of his work. Most of the food served at these lunches is quite rich, but there is always a wide variety of cold cuts. If Bob has decided that he is going to eat only 3 meat exchanges on a day when he is supposed to go to a buffet lunch, how many cold cuts (size: 4½″ x ⅛″) can he eat? Circle one:

3

6    3    2    4

5. In Week Two, your diet, aside from those foods which you may have in any quantity at any time during the program, will come com-

pletely from the meat and vegetable A groups. (We'll cover the
vegetable A exchanges later in this
chapter.) In all, you will be allowed 49 meat exchanges for the
first week. If you were to formu-
late a diet allowing an equal number of meat exchanges over a
seven-day period, you would give
yourself a total of _____ meat exchanges a day.

7

6. Suppose that on the last day
of this week of your diet you discover that you have eaten only 40
meat exchanges. This would mean
that you would be allowed to eat
_____ meat exchanges on the last
day of the week, because you are
allowed 49 meat exchanges for the
entire week.

9

7. Circle the number of meat exchanges that you may have during
Week Two.

49                56      42      39      49

Here is the list of meat exchange equivalents that
we have worked with previously, and a menu comprised

of foods taken exclusively from the meat group. Check each item on the menu list against the Meat Exchange Equivalents list and write the number of exchanges that item is worth in the spaces provided. Remember that each item on the Meat Exchange Equivalents list is equal to one exchange when used in the amounts provided, but that the menu list will show amounts greater than those on the equivalents list.

---

## MEAT EXCHANGE EQUIVALENTS
### *Each Item Equals One Meat Exchange*

| | |
|---|---|
| Any meat or poultry (medium-fat) | 1 ounce |
| Cold cuts (4½″ x ⅛″) | 1 slice |
| Frankfurter (8–9 per pound) | 1 |
| Egg | 1 |
| Any fresh fish | 2 ounces |
| Canned fish | ¼ cup |
| Shellfish (shrimp, clams, oysters, etc.) | 5 small |
| Any cheese * | 1 ounce |
| Cottage cheese | ¼ cup |

* *Except cream cheese.*

FISH (FRESH OR FROZEN)

  8 ounces haddock equals _____ exchanges.

MEAT

  8 ounces liver equals _____ exchanges.
  6 ounces lamb equals _____ exchanges.

**POULTRY**

16 ounces (1 pound) chicken equals _____ exchanges.

**CANNED FISH**

½ cup (¼ + ¼ = ½) crab equals _____ exchanges.
½ cup tuna equals _____ exchanges.

**MISCELLANEOUS**

4 frankfurters equal _____ exchanges.
6 eggs equal _____ exchanges.
¼ cup cottage cheese equals _____ exchanges.

Correct answers to the above questions appear below and on the following page.

**FISH (FRESH OR FROZEN)**

8 ounces haddock equals 4 exchanges.

**MEAT**

8 ounces liver equals 8 exchanges.
6 ounces lamb equals 6 exchanges.

**POULTRY**

16 ounces (1 pound) chicken equals 16 exchanges.

**CANNED FISH**

½ cup (¼ + ¼ = ½) crab equals 2 exchanges.
½ cup tuna equals 2 exchanges.

**MISCELLANEOUS**

4 frankfurters equal 4 exchanges.

93

6 eggs equal 6 exchanges.
¼ cup cottage cheese equals 1 exchange.

If you made any mistakes, be sure to find out where you went wrong before you continue.

Below is the same Meat Exchange Equivalents list that we worked with in the last problem, and another menu list. Find out how many exchanges each item on the list is worth. Then find out how many meat exchanges are represented by the entire list. Again, keep in mind that each item on the Meat Exchange Equivalents list is equal to one meat exchange when used in the amounts shown, but that the foods on the menu list will usually be in greater amounts than those on the equivalents list.

### MEAT EXCHANGE EQUIVALENTS

*Each Item Equals One Meat Exchange*

| | |
|---|---|
| Any meat or poultry (medium-fat) | 1 ounce |
| Cold cuts (4½″ x ⅛″) | 1 slice |
| Frankfurter (8–9 per pound) | 1 |
| Egg | 1 |
| Any fresh fish | 2 ounces |
| Canned fish | ¼ cup |
| Shellfish (shrimp, clams, oysters, etc.) | 5 small |
| Any cheese * | 1 ounce |
| Cottage cheese | ¼ cup |

* *Except cream cheese.*

FISH (FRESH OR FROZEN)
>   6 ounces mackerel equals _____ exchanges.
>   6 ounces halibut equals _____ exchanges.

MEAT
>   16 ounces ground beef equals _____ exchanges.

POULTRY
>   10 ounces chicken equals _____ exchanges.

CANNED FISH
>   ½ cup tuna equals _____ exchanges.
>   ½ cup salmon equals _____ exchanges.

MISCELLANEOUS
>   1 dozen eggs equal _____ exchanges.
>   ¼ cup cottage cheese equals _____ exchanges.

WRITE TOTAL NUMBER OF EXCHANGES _____.

Correct answers appear below and on the following page.

FISH (FRESH OR FROZEN)
>   6 ounces mackerel equals 3 meat exchanges.
>   6 ounces halibut equals 3 meat exchanges.

MEAT
>   16 ounces ground beef equals 16 meat exchanges.

POULTRY
>   10 ounces chicken equals 10 meat exchanges.

CANNED FISH

½ cup tuna equals 2 meat exchanges.

½ cup salmon equals 2 meat exchanges.

MISCELLANEOUS

1 dozen eggs equals 12 meat exchanges.

¼ cup cottage cheese equals 1 meat exchange.

TOTAL: 49 meat exchanges.

Again, if you have made any mistakes, find out where you went wrong before you continue.

## THE VEGETABLE A LIST

In addition to the 49 meat exchanges you are allowed during Week Two, you can also eat unlimited amounts from the Vegetable A List. In fact, throughout the diet and for as long as you continue on this plan, you may eat unlimited amounts from this group, *as long as you do not cook them.* If you prefer cooked vegetables to raw, the amount you may eat is more restricted, as you will learn.

On the following pages you will find a series of problems designed to familiarize you with the foods on the Vegetable A List. Remember to cover the answer column.

1. Vegetables included in the Vegetable A List have very little

food value. That is, the content of fats, carbohydrates, and proteins and calories in these foods is so low that it is considered negligible. The fact that these foods have very lit-

food value

tle f ___ v ___ is what makes it possible for you to eat an unlimited amount of these foods so long as you don't cook them.

2. You may eat an unlimited amount of foods from the Vegetable A List so long as you eat them

raw

(*cooked/raw*).

unlimited

3. You may eat (*unlimited/limited*) amounts of foods from the Vegetable A List so long as you do not cook them, but if you cannot tolerate uncooked vegetables, you must limit your intake of these foods to *one cup per meal.*

4. If you choose to cook your A vegetables, then you must limit

one

your intake of these foods to o ___ cup per meal per day.

three

5. Assuming you are going to eat three meals a day, and that you are going to cook all of your A vegetables, you would then be eating a total of _____ cups of cooked A vegetables per day.

increase

6. If vegetable A foods consist primarily of calories and water, and cooking them removes a great deal of water, you (*decrease/increase*) the concentration of calories in the food. This is why you are allowed only one cup of cooked vegetables per meal, but unlimited uncooked vegetable A's.

7. Circle the amount of cooked A vegetables that you may have at *each meal each day:*

1 cup                    1½ cups          3 cups          1 cup
                                    ½ cup

As long as you eat foods from the vegetable A group raw, you may eat just as much of them as you can hold. Just remember: the more you eat of these foods, the more water your body will tend to retain. But if you feel you absolutely must have lots of these vegetables to stave off hunger, feel free to indulge yourself. In the next few weeks you will lose whatever excess water you retain.

On this page you will find a list of all the vegetable A's. The next set of questions will be based on this list, so you may find it necessary to refer back to it for your answers.

## VEGETABLE A LIST

| | | |
|---|---|---|
| Artichokes | Chicory | Pepper, green |
| Asparagus | Cucumbers | Radishes |
| Broccoli | Eggplant | Rhubarb |
| Brussels sprouts | Escarole | Sauerkraut |
| Cabbage | Lettuce | String beans, young |
| Cauliflower | Mushrooms | Summer squash |
| Celery | Okra | Tomatoes |

### GREENS

| | | | |
|---|---|---|---|
| Beet | Collard | Kale | Spinach |
| Chard | Dandelion | Mustard | Turnip |

1. Asparagus is a food on the Vegetable A List. As long as you eat asparagus raw, you may have (*limited/unlimited*) amounts of this food.

unlimited

2. Foods on the Vegetable A List are limited to one cup per meal when they are (*cooked/uncooked*).

cooked

99

one cup

3.   Cauliflower is on the Vegetable A List. If you wanted to have cooked cauliflower with your dinner, you could have (*one/two/three*) cup(s).

4.   Here is a list of four vegetables. Which one is not on the Vegetable A List? Refer back to the list if necessary.
a. cabbage
b. lettuce

c. potatoes

c. potatoes
d. tomatoes

5.   Here is a list of several vegetables. Look over the list, compare it to the Vegetable A List, and check off the ones you may eat in unlimited quantities as long as they are uncooked:

cucumber
eggplant
rhubarb

☐ cucumber          ☐ rhubarb
☐ eggplant          ☐ green peas
☐ carrots           ☐ pumpkin

Every long-term dieter knows the vegetable A's. We are using them as fillers for now, but you'll be off the celery-and-lettuce circuit soon. If these vegetables irritate your intestines, cooking them might make all the difference in the world. (But remember: if you cook vegetable A's, you are limited to one cup per meal.)

You may use a dab of any commercial low-calorie dressing to liven up the flavor a bit, but don't get carried away—diet dressings still have lots of calories and can be very fattening if you use too much. A tablespoon is about the right amount. Better still, use the Zero Salad Dressing described on page 230.

Keep in mind that not *all* vegetables are included on the Vegetable A List. If you are dining out and you're not sure if the vegetables being served are on the unlimited list, pass up the questionable foods.

On the following page you will find a tally sheet for keeping track of how many meat exchanges you eat each day. You needn't keep a record of the vegetables if you eat them raw, but if you cook them, include them on the tally.

Record the number of meat exchanges that you have for each meal or snack during Week Two in the spaces provided below. Total each day as you go along and try to keep the number of meat exchanges per day as close to 7 as possible, since you have a total of 49 meat exchanges per week. Do not exceed this total. And try to avoid having to go hungry on the last day of the week.

## MEAT EXCHANGES

*1st Day  2nd Day  3rd Day  4th Day  5th Day  6th Day  7th Day*

TOTALS

Record the number of cups of cooked A vegetables that you have each day during Week Two of your diet in the spaces below. Remember that you are limited to 1 cup per meal per day.

## CUPS OF COOKED A VEGETABLES

*1st Day  2nd Day  3rd Day  4th Day  5th Day  6th Day  7th Day*

TOTALS

The total grams of carbohydrates, proteins, and fats per exchange in your Week Two diet each day are:

102

| | Carbohydrates | Proteins | Fats |
|---|---|---|---|
| Meat (7 per day) | 0 | 49 | 35 |
| Vegetable A's (unlimited if uncooked) | 0 — | 0 — | 0 — |
| TOTAL GRAMS: | 0 | 49 | 35 |
| TOTAL CALORIES: | 0 | 196 | 315 = 511 per day |

## WEEK TWO EXERCISE

From Week Two on, your exercise is going to be rigorous enough so that you'll require a brief warm-up before you begin. What you will be doing, basically, is taking five minutes to let your body know that you are preparing to put some strain on your heart, circulation, and muscles; this warning period will allow your pulse rate to accelerate gradually rather than in a sudden and steep incline. It will also loosen your muscles so that you don't experience aches and pains as a result of your activity.

Here's what you need to do:

—Six stretching exercises. Stretch your arms up toward the ceiling as far as you can, then bend at the waist (knees straight) and stretch your arms toward the floor. Touch the floor if you can.

103

—Six arm-swings. Rotate your arms in large circles, swinging all the way from the shoulder.

—Walk around briskly for two minutes, going faster and faster until you break into a jog. Gradually raise your knees higher and higher.

—End up with a few more stretches.

I mention specific numbers of exercises, but once you are accustomed to warming up, you'll know how much you need before you feel loose, comfortable, and ready to begin.

When you finish your activity session, cool down in exactly the same way that you warmed up, repeating the exercises. Try to *feel* your system slowing down, your heart and circulation returning to normal.

Five minutes after exercise you should be breathing normally, with your pulse rate down to under 120 beats per minute. Within ten minutes your pulse should be under 100. If this is not the case, you are *working too hard* and must back up one week in your exercise program.

Again let me remind you: if at any time you feel dizzy, light-headed, or nauseated, stop exercising, but continue to walk slowly. Take your pulse. If you find that you are continually interrupting your exercise because of these symptoms, notify your doctor. For someone exercising daily at the gentle rate prescribed here, such reactions are unusual, and you should find out as soon as possible what the trouble is.

*Never* exercise when you have a cold, fever, or any infection of your entire system. If you do become ill, wait until you are healthy again and go back one week in your exercise schedule, so you can rebuild your endurance.

If you've chosen to exercise outdoors, and the temperature is below thirty-two degrees or above ninety degrees, cut your exercise time *in half for one week*, until you are acclimated. A few seasons ago, several of the San Francisco 49ers were hospitalized after a game with the Dolphins in Miami, not because of injuries but because they were not accustomed to Florida's intense heat. And although your activity sessions won't be nearly as strenuous as a pro football game, I think it's also fair to assume that you aren't in anything like the physical condition of a professional athlete!

If you should vacation in an altitude above 5,000 feet, again exercise at *half your rate* for a week until you are used to breathing air with less oxygen. Then gradually return to your normal schedule.

Whatever adaptations you may have to make in your exercise schedule, continue with the regular diet for that week.

Before our discussion of Week Two, let me remind you of our general guidelines for this and every week:

—Monitor your pulse rate.

—Warm up before and cool down after each physical-exercise session.

—Do not exercise when you are ill.

Many of my patients are in a hurry to get the job done. Remember that sound physical conditioning takes time. Have patience, don't overdo it, and all the benefits of a fine, healthy body will be yours.

## YOUR FIRST PHYSICAL ACTIVITY TEST

From now on, it will be necessary to divide you up into bikers and walkers (although you are all dieters, please!). Whether you've chosen to walk or bike, you will achieve the same level of physical fitness at the end of the program, but you will be working toward different goals in terms of both time and distance.

I believe that one of the keys to my patients' success is the flexibility of the exercise plan. Not that you can avoid hard work—you *cannot*—but you are never forced to undertake any exercise that overtaxes you. When your heart rate indicates you are ready to go on to harder work, that is when you go on, and not before. So you can never abandon the exercise completely, moaning, "It was too hard for me!" Remember: *you* are making the decisions here; I am not.

To test yourself, you need a watch with a second

hand. If there is no track in your neighborhood, just get in your car, drive a mile, note a landmark at that point and drive home. You have now charted a standard two-mile course for yourself.

Do you remember how to take your own pulse? (See p. 55.) Remember, it is essential that your heartbeat *reach the training range without exceeding it.*

## Bicycling

After six days of Week One exercise—cycling indoors on a stationary bike or riding outdoors—you are probably able to travel two miles in ten minutes. If you cannot, keep trying to achieve that goal this week and take your test seven days from now. Don't be discouraged. You are not in a race. You are simply trying to become healthy at a pace that is natural for you.

If you *can* pedal two miles in ten minutes after six days, on the seventh day of Week One try to travel two miles in *eight* minutes without pushing your heart past its training rate. If you can achieve this goal without exceeding your training limit, then you have your second week's regimen: travel two miles in eight minutes for the next five days.

If you cannot complete the two miles in eight minutes (or, to put it another way, two four-minute miles), return to the Week One goal and travel two miles in ten minutes for five more days. Don't be discouraged. The

107

Week Two goal is demanding for a beginner, and it may be a while coming. *Do not push yourself* too hard to get there. Take as much time as *you* need to work up to that speed, and keep checking your pulse rate every time you exercise. In another week or so you *will* achieve the Week Two goal, and the rest will come much more easily. Don't worry about falling behind. If you work up to this goal in two or more weeks, you will find yourself surpassing test goals later on, and skipping ahead. So do only what you *can* do; your Week Two doesn't have to be the same as someone else's (*except on the diet!*).

The Week One exercise is sometimes so successful for a patient that the test for Week Two does not even push his heart up to the allowable training rate. If your heartbeat is more than 10 percent below the lower limit of your range, wait until the next day and try to go two and *a half* miles in *ten* minutes. If you can do so safely, make that your Week Two program.

This test will determine what you are going to be doing for the next five days. On the sixth day you are going to rest, and on the seventh take the test for Week Three, which we'll talk about at the beginning of our Week Three chapter.

### Walking

After six days of walking, you can probably cover two miles in 40 minutes. If you cannot do so, then that is still your goal. Otherwise, you will test yourself now—at the end of Week One—to see if you can walk your two miles in less than 40 minutes. If you are able to achieve the two miles in a half hour, that's terrific; two miles in 30 minutes is your Week Two goal. Walk at that rate for the next five days.

Trying to walk faster on this test day than you have in the past six days may cause your heart to beat at an unacceptable rate. If so, slow down tomorrow, even if this puts you back to your previous accomplishment of two miles in 40 minutes. Then, for the next five days, walk *at the best rate your heart allows* between 30 and 40 minutes. If you covered the distance in 34 minutes on this test day, don't be lazy and let yourself walk at 40 minutes. Maintain your test-day time for the five days of Week Two.

As long as you are completing the course in 40 minutes or less, you are continuing to strengthen your heart, your body, and your endurance, and you will certainly be able to cut your time down to 30 minutes on the next test day.

On the other hand, you may have found that the test walk did not even push your heart up to a training rate. This means that you are already fit enough to accomplish two miles in 30 minutes without trouble. If this is so, try to walk two and *a half* miles in 37½ minutes. You will not only be walking faster than you were in Week One, but you will be walking farther. (Remember: this two-and-a-half-mile goal is only for those who are not sufficiently taxed by the basic Week Two goal of two miles in 30 minutes.)

You've now settled upon a goal for Week Two. Work at it for the next five days. Be sure to rest on the sixth.

One more tip for you walkers: get a pair of comfortable walking shoes. You may think your everyday shoes are quite comfortable, but you haven't done this much exercise in them before, and I doubt that traditional hard leather shoes will give you the best support. Jogging shoes are best, but any sport shoe will be better than your wingtips, gentlemen, or your wedgies, ladies.

One final remark, for both bikers and walkers: if you can accomplish the Week Two goal by the end of the second week, you should easily achieve fitness by the end of this program. If it takes you an extra week or two to reach this goal—which is not at all uncommon—don't be discouraged. It will take you a little longer to get into shape, but you will notice even more remarkable improvements in your health and energy when you *do* succeed.

## YOUR REACTION TO THE WEEK TWO DIET

After seven days on a meat and vegetable A diet you should have a good idea of how these two groups make you feel. My patients' responses usually fall into three general categories.

For most patients, Week Two is a good week. They

register weight losses from 5 to 15 pounds, and sometimes more. These patients become walking advertisements for our clinic, because they tell everyone, "Yes, I am dieting and I feel terrific. I'm on top of the world."

If you feel great this week, take that as a warning. You benefit from a diet with *limited carbohydrates,* so when fruit (Week Three) and bread (Week Seven) are added to your diet, your weight loss may suddenly come to a halt. But if it does, you'll learn how to get back on your weight-loss schedule in the Week Three and Week Seven chapters.

Even though Week Two's diet has left you feeling great, let me warn you not to plan on staying with Week Two until you have lost all the weight you want. Like the Week One starter diet, Week Two's diet *should not be extended longer than seven days.* The purpose of this plan is to take off weight easily, safely, and permanently. The Week Two diet is not a safe long-term diet; it is a temporary diet plan and should be used only in that way.

Now that you know you react well to a minimum of carbohydrates, you should realize how important your physical activity is. Although I want you to stay away from carbohydrates for the time being, it's unrealistic—as well as unhealthy—to expect yourself to give them up *forever.* The only solution, then, is to change your body chemistry through exercise. Only then will you be able to make peace with carbohydrates.

❖          ❖          ❖

A few patients begin to feel bad after two or three days of Week Two's meat and vegetable diet. Their bodies are telling them they will never benefit from a limited-carbohydrate diet. If you are in this category, don't get upset. Continue with the plan. In only a few more days we will be introducing fruit, with all its carbohydrates. Your discomfort this week is probably caused by dehydration and a slight ketosis (an abnormal burning of body fats), and the symptoms are usually quite mild. However, eating more vegetables will help these symptoms disappear.

Chances are, if you are not a heavy eater (as indicated in the quizzes in the chapter titled "Why Are *You* Fat?"), you suffer from a severe lack of physical activity. You need carbohydrates to feel good. But those same carbohydrates are causing your weight gain. The only way out of this trap is to increase the number of calories you burn each day through physical activity and greater Lean Body Mass.

Some patients experience *neither* of these noticeable reactions. If you felt perfectly normal during this week, that tells us as much about your body as the other two more extreme responses. Meat and vegetables present no obstacles for you, and you are not a carbohydrate addict. Your problems, if any, will show up in future weeks. Meanwhile, continue with the test diet and activity schedules. You are doing fine.

## WEEK TWO PROBLEMS

Week Two will be tougher than the first week. You will have more exchange-dieting material to learn, and your physical activity won't be getting any easier. That is why I want to take some time here to try to answer all your questions. After Week Two, each of the remaining five weeks on this plan will be easier and easier.

For most of you, your scale will be giving you reward enough. The Week Two diet contains primarily proteins and fats, with a minimum of fattening carbohydrates, so many patients experience a loss of 10 to 20 pounds or more. I am sure you will find such weight loss exciting. But no matter how much the scale *says* you lost, it is highly unlikely that you will lose more than 10 pounds of fat in two weeks. It is more likely that your actual fat loss will be 8½ pounds at most, the rest being water loss.

Remember these first two weeks in the days to come, when you seem to be losing weight more slowly. The fact is, you will still be losing approximately as much fat, but the loss will not show up on your scale because you may begin retaining water in the near future.

Within these forty-nine days, your weight loss will not proceed in a straight, downward path. There are great shifts of water in the body and it is not unusual for a person to gain or lose 5 pounds in any given day. We call that "tide going in" and "tide going out." When the tide comes in, almost nothing you do will result in weight loss and

113

you could even show a weight gain. There is nothing more frustrating for me than an anguished patient who has stuck rigidly to the diet and exercised faithfully, standing in front of me in tears because, despite everything, he or she has gained two pounds.

You *cannot* let yourself be frustrated by the shift in water. You are *still losing fat no matter what your scale shows*. It is simply disguised by the water gain. You will have to wait, but your fat loss *will* become evident in the course of the plan.

In these first two weeks, you may develop high blood fats. If you visit your doctor during this time, he may find a higher cholesterol level than usual.

Don't worry. This change in blood fats is only temporary. Furthermore, you are doing a good amount of exercise for the first time in years, and that's very good for battling cholesterol levels.

However, if you are concerned about cholesterol, during Week Two choose primarily from the fish and fowl groups and keep the amount of meat, eggs, and cheese you eat at a minimum. A patient gave our clinic this message in needlepoint, and we ask our cholesterol watchers to remember it:

> If it swims, it is better than if it flies. If it flies, it is better than if it walks. If it walks, it is certainly better than if it lies there—like an egg.

High levels of uric acid are one of the known causes of gout, but this has never been a problem for us. Though my patients do show high uric-acid levels during Week Two, *not one* has exhibited or complained of symptoms of gout. However, to dilute the acid somewhat during this week, drink large amounts of liquids—*at least eight glasses per day*, preferably more.

You may drink decaffeinated coffee, tea, diet drinks containing less than 3 calories per eight-ounce bottle (read the label carefully), bouillon, and water. Besides diluting uric-acid concentration, all this liquid will also push your body closer to its saturation point and you will begin giving up water in your urine. As I mentioned at the end of Week One, if water retention is a problem for you, stick to *salt-free* liquids as much as possible. The more of them you drink, the sooner your real weight loss will begin to show.

A small number of people find their weight loss dramatically impeded by hormones, either their own or those taken as medication. *Women beginning this diet one week before their menstrual period frequently fail to lose weight.*

In the week preceding the menses, large amounts of salt- and water-retaining hormones are manufactured by the ovaries. These hormones are efficient at holding salt and water, so they will disguise your fat loss. But you have lost fat nonetheless. Three or four days after the beginning of your period, these hormones will disappear and a very rapid weight loss will occur.

Women who are just beginning to take female hormones, either as birth-control pills or to modify the symptoms of menopause, will encounter the same difficulty.

Please try to keep in mind that your body can hold only so much water before it must flush that water out of your system. Water retention can continue for as long as four weeks, and no weight loss may show up during that time. However, once the spill takes place, you will lose weight in a steady and consistent manner. By the time you reach Week Seven, you will have observed the same results as those whose weight loss showed from Week One on.

A few people also react to low-calorie diets by excreting an antidiuretic hormone from the pituitary gland. Known as ADH, this hormone is a powerful water-retainer and will immediately block the body's attempt to lose weight. ADH sees to it that water replaces every bit of fat that you burn off. Occasionally a pound of fat will be replaced by *more* than a pound of water, so that a person actually shows a weight gain during the first few weeks of the plan. I have seen patients go as long as twenty-two days before they begin to show weight loss. This can be terribly discouraging and, to be honest, it has caused some people to quit the program.

*Don't quit.*

Every patient with the problem of ADH who has hung on until his weight loss begins to show has gone on to conclude the program successfully.

Another problem that arises during the second week is something my patients call constipation. *Constipation* is a very specific medical term describing infrequent stools that are hard and are painful to excrete. This is *not* the

116

situation our patients describe. Rather, they simply find that they are no longer having bowel movements every day. Two or three times a week is average—and sufficient —during Week Two. The stools are well formed and soft (and not painful to excrete); this is simply a manifestation of the fact that you are eating food with little residue.

There is no law in nature demanding a bowel movement every day. That is a rumor propagated by people who make a very good living selling laxatives. You don't need to use a laxative during Week Two, and in fact I wish you wouldn't; often they can be irritating to your intestines.

# Week Three

## WEEK THREE EXERCISE

Your diet throughout the entire seven weeks of our plan is totally regimented. You are allowed a fixed, specific amount of food no matter what. Only at the end of the forty-nine days will you be able to devise your own individual diet, based on your knowledge of exchange dieting and what you've learned about the effects of each food group on your system.

With the exercise plan, however, I'm going to be letting go of you a little sooner. Right now, in fact. At this point your exercise plan is going to become so individual that it will be impossible for me to continue discussing "the plan." There is no longer just one plan. From now on, your weekly goals will be dictated, not by me, but by your body's capabilities. Monitoring your heartbeat rate is going to be more important than ever, since you will be relying on your heart to tell you when you are ready to work harder, or if you've skipped ahead too fast and need to slow down for a few days. But before I explain this procedure in more detail, let me give you some good news.

Now that you have achieved the Week Two goal (and you wouldn't be reading this chapter if you hadn't), you are no longer going to work at increasing your *rate* of exercise. If you are biking, you are now traveling at fifteen miles per hour. Walkers are traveling at four miles per hour. For both bikers *and* walkers, *this is the fastest rate you will ever need to go.* From now on, every week you will increase the *distance* you bike or walk, but at the same time you will also be increasing the amount of *time* you allow yourself for covering that distance. A lot more hard work lies ahead, but the fact is you have accomplished the first major goal of the exercise program. So relax for a moment while I explain what happens next.

It will now be up to you to fix your own goals for each week. Some of you, however, will progress at a more or less average rate, and those who do can use the following goals as a rule of thumb:

### BIKERS

| Week | Distance | Time | Rate |
|------|----------|------|------|
| 1 | 2 miles | 10 minutes | 12 mph |
| 2 | 2 miles | 8 minutes | 15 mph |
| 3 | 2½ miles | 10 minutes | 15 mph |
| 4 | 3½ miles | 14 minutes | 15 mph |
| 5 | 4 miles | 16 minutes | 15 mph |
| 6 | 5 miles | 20 minutes | 15 mph |
| 7 | 6 miles | 24 minutes | 15 mph |

### WALKERS

| Week | Distance | Time | Rate |
|------|----------|------|------|
| 1 | 2 miles | 40 minutes | 3 mph |
| 2 | 2 miles | 30 minutes | 4 mph |
| 3 | 2½ miles | 37½ minutes | 4 mph |
| 4 | 2½ miles | 37½ minutes | 4 mph |
| 5 | 3 miles | 45 minutes | 4 mph |
| 6 | 3½ miles | 52½ minutes | 4 mph |
| 7 | 4 miles | 60 minutes | 4 mph |

But the chart is only a guideline. What I am about to explain about setting your own goals applies to *every-*

*one*: in the weeks intervening between Week Two and Week Seven, you will decide how much you need to do on the basis of your body's reactions. Keeping your heartbeat within the training range that's safe for you is much more important than conforming to these rough guidelines. That is why only you can map out, week by week, what your activity goal will be.

As you can see on the charts, the ultimate Week Seven goals are:

BIKERS: 6 miles in 24 minutes

WALKERS: 4 miles in 60 minutes

These goals are *not* flexible. Once you have reached them, you will continue exercising 24 or 60 minutes a day, every day, for the rest of your life. So as you can see, there's no rush getting there. If you reach the Week Seven goal in Week Four, congratulations. You will simply burn off pounds and achieve fitness faster than most. If the forty-ninth day arrives and you are still weeks away from achieving Week Seven's goal, don't feel defeated. What matters is that you try your *very best* every single day of every week between now and the end of the forty-nine days. And doing your best requires that you learn to listen to what your body tells you.

Immediately after an exercise period, monitor your body's reactions. Do you feel especially good as soon as you stop? If so, test yourself the very next day to see if

121

you can go half a mile farther without exceeding the limits of your heart's training range. *Don't* waste an entire week repeating a distance you can already achieve easily.

Remember, every time you increase your distance you must also allow yourself more time to cover it.

WALKERS: Every time you add half a mile to your distance, allow yourself 7½ more minutes.

BIKERS: Every time you add half a mile to your distance, allow yourself an additional 2 minutes.

If increasing your distance exhausts you and causes your heartbeat to exceed the training level, do not hesitate to drop back and continue covering whatever distance you *can* safely achieve. After a few more days test yourself again to see if there is any change.

Here's what you should do right now:

### Bikers

You are now able to travel 2 miles in 8 minutes. On your Week Three test day, then, try to go 2½ miles in 10 minutes. If you can do so safely, that is your exercise plan for the next five days. After *three* days, however, try increasing your distance (and time) slightly. If your heartbeat speeds up too fast, continue doing 2½ miles in

10 minutes for the full five days. Then test yourself again on a greater distance.

If you cannot go 2½ miles in 10 minutes, continue doing 2 miles in 8 minutes for three more days, then test yourself again. *Gradually* increase your speed—perhaps a quarter of a mile at a time, instead of half a mile —until you can cover 2½ miles in 10 minutes. Then begin the process again, this time aiming at the Week Four guideline.

## Walkers

You are now able to travel 2 miles in 30 minutes. On your Week Three test day, then, try to go 2½ miles in 37½ minutes. If you can do so safely, that is your exercise plan for the next five days. This is a difficult goal, so don't rush past it. Give your body some time to adjust to this increased effort. Once you have passed this goal, you will probably progress quickly.

If you cannot go 2½ miles in 37½ minutes, don't be surprised or discouraged. As you can see on the chart, we allow two full weeks to reach this goal, and some people require even more time. So don't rush. Continue doing 2 miles in 30 minutes for three more days. Then test yourself again. *Gradually* increase your speed—perhaps a quarter or even an eighth of a mile at a time instead of half a mile—until you can cover 2½ miles in 37½ minutes (this may well take you until the end of Week Four).

Spend a few days at that speed. Then begin the process again, this time aiming at the Week Five guideline.

*Rule of thumb for bikers and walkers.* Whenever you manage to improve slightly, stick with your new time and distance for a few days, then try a little harder.

Obviously, this part of the program relies on being honest with yourself. You must work as hard as your body will let you. Do not work harder, but don't go easy on yourself either.

If you are persistent, you cannot fail with this plan. There is no place *to* fail, because you are not racing toward a deadline. You will succeed when you succeed. For many of you, success will come in Week Seven. For some it will be sooner and for others it will be later. But it will come, eventually, for everyone.

## WEEK THREE DIET

Your diet for Week Three will still include the meat and vegetable exchanges you were allowed during Week Two. You will be adding 14 exchanges per week from the fruit list. Fruit is pure carbohydrate, so many of you can expect a marked reaction when you add this food to your test diet. Pay close attention to fluctuations in weight, hunger, and energy level.

In the next pages you will learn exactly how to integrate fruit into your diet. Remember the rules and don't look at the printed answer until you've given your own. Be sure to respond to all the questions.

In the section on meat exchanges you learned that all meat exchanges have the same number of fats, proteins, and calories per exchange. Similarly, every fruit exchange has the same number of carbohydrates and calories as every other fruit exchange.

1. A fruit exchange contains 10 grams of carbohydrate and 40 calories. One small apple and one small orange are both equal to one fruit exchange. Does this mean that you could eat a small apple instead of a small orange?

YES

YES        NO

2. A fruit exchange contains 10 grams of carbohydrate. Since there are 4 calories in every gram of carbohydrate, there must be_____ calories in every fruit exchange.

40

3. Circle the number of grams of carbohydrate contained in one fruit exchange:

10

12        9        10        40

125

4. Circle the number of calories in one fruit exchange:

40                10     4     40     0

5. Your diet for Week Three consists of the same foods you have eaten during the first two weeks, plus 14 fruit exchanges per week. If you wanted to arrange your menu so that you would eat an equal number of fruit exchanges each day of the week, you would

2        eat _____ fruit exchanges each day.

6. So far, your diet is composed

49       of _____ meat exchanges a week,

14       _____ fruit exchanges a week, and an unlimited amount of uncooked vegetable A's (or one cup of cooked vegetable A's per meal).

Following is a list of all the foods on the fruit exchange list. Each food in the amount listed is equal to *one fruit exchange.* For the next set of questions, you will need to refer back to this list.

## FRUIT EXCHANGE EQUIVALENTS
### *Each Item Equals One Fruit Exchange*

| | |
|---|---|
| Apple | 1 small (2″ in diam.) |
| Applesauce | ½ cup |
| Apricots, dried | 4 halves |
| Apricots, fresh | 2 medium |
| Banana | ½ small |
| Berries (strawberries blackberries, raspberries) | 1 cup |
| Blueberries | ⅔ cup |
| Cantaloupe | ¼ (6″ in diam.) |
| Cherries | 10 large |
| Dates | 2 |
| Figs, dried | 1 small |
| Figs, fresh | 2 large |
| Grapefruit | ½ small |
| Grapefruit juice | ½ cup |
| Grape juice | ¼ cup |
| Grapes | 12 |
| Honeydew melon | ⅛ (7″ in diam.) |
| Mango | ½ small |
| Orange | 1 small |
| Orange juice | ½ cup |
| Papaya | ⅓ medium |
| Peach | 1 medium |
| Pear | 1 small |
| Pineapple | ½ cup |
| Pineapple juice | ⅓ cup |
| Plums | 2 medium |
| Prunes, dried | 2 medium |
| Raisins | 2 tbsp. |
| Tangerine | 1 large |
| Watermelon | 1 cup |

You are permitted to eat *any* fruit you can think of during Week Three, even if it is not specified on the Fruit Exchange Equivalents list. Just choose a listed fruit that is similar to the unlisted fruit you want to eat— a peach, say, is roughly similar to a nectarine, so one medium-sized nectarine would equal one fruit exchange, even though nectarines are not on the list.

1. Here are five fruits from the fruit exchange list. Write in the amount required to make each fruit equal to one exchange.

| | | |
|---|---|---|
| 10 large | Cherries | _____ |
| 2 medium | Plums | _____ |
| 1 small | Orange | _____ |
| 1 small | Apple | _____ |
| 1 cup | Berries | _____ |

2. Check off the fruits that are *not* equal to one fruit exchange. Pay close attention to quantities.

|  | |
|---|---|
| | ½ cup applesauce |
| 24 grapes | 24 grapes |
| | ½ cup grapefruit juice |
| 3 tbsp. raisins | 3 tablespoons raisins |
| | 1 cup watermelon |

3. Below are two lists, "A" and "B." Remembering that you are allowed a total of 14 fruit exchanges, look over these two lists and decide which one is appropriate for this diet; that is, which one does not exceed the limitation of 14 fruit exchanges.

LIST A

|   | | |
|---|---|---|
| 3 | 3 small apples = _____ exchanges |
| 6 | 6 small oranges = _____ exchanges |
| 2 | 1 cup pineapple = _____ exchanges |
| 3 | 6 medium plums = _____ exchanges |
| 14 total | _____ TOTAL |

LIST B

|   | | |
|---|---|---|
| 4 | 2 mangoes = _____ exchanges |
| 11 | 11 small apples = _____ exchanges |
| 15 total | _____ TOTAL |

On the following page you will find a tally sheet similar to the one you used during Week Two. This tally sheet provides space for you to record the number of fruit exchanges you eat at each snack or meal for each day during the next week, along with the meat and vegetable A exchanges.

Remember, to ensure that you don't exceed the 49-meat-exchange limitation per week, try to keep close to 7 meat exchanges per day.

Similarly, to ensure that you don't have to give up eating fruit on any day, try to keep your daily fruit exchanges as close to 2 as possible.

Record the number of meat exchanges that you use for each meal or snack during Week Three in the spaces below. Total each day as you go along, and try to keep the number of your daily exchanges as close to 7 as possible.

## MEAT EXCHANGES

| 1st Day | 2nd Day | 3rd Day | 4th Day | 5th Day | 6th Day | 7th Day |
|---------|---------|---------|---------|---------|---------|---------|
|         |         |         |         |         |         |         |
|         |         |         |         |         |         |         |
|         |         |         |         |         |         |         |
|         |         |         |         |         |         |         |
|         |         |         |         |         |         |         |

TOTALS

Record the number of 1-cup portions of cooked vegetable A's that you have each day for Week Three in the spaces below. Remember that if you cook your vegetable A's you are limited to 3 cups per day.

### CUPS OF COOKED A VEGETABLES

| 1st Day | 2nd Day | 3rd Day | 4th Day | 5th Day | 6th Day | 7th Day |
|---------|---------|---------|---------|---------|---------|---------|
|         |         |         |         |         |         |         |
|         |         |         |         |         |         |         |

TOTALS

Record the number of fruit exchanges that you have at each meal or snack during the next week in the spaces below. Remember that you are allowed 14 fruit exchanges per week, so try to keep your fruit exchanges as close to 2 per day as possible.

### FRUIT EXCHANGES

| 1st Day | 2nd Day | 3rd Day | 4th Day | 5th Day | 6th Day | 7th Day |
|---------|---------|---------|---------|---------|---------|---------|
|         |         |         |         |         |         |         |
|         |         |         |         |         |         |         |

TOTALS

During Week Three you are receiving the following grams of carbohydrates, proteins, and fats in each day's exchanges:

|  | Carbohydrates | Proteins | Fats |
|---|---|---|---|
| Meat (7 per day) | 0 | 49 | 35 |
| Vegetable A's (unlimited if uncooked) | 0 | 0 | 0 |
| Fruit (2 per day) | 20 | 0 | 0 |
| TOTAL GRAMS: | 20 | 49 | 35 |
| TOTAL CALORIES: | 80 | 196 | 315=591 per day |

## WEEK THREE PROBLEMS

Everyone eats the same food in Week Three, but many people have opposite reactions. How are *you* feeling this week?

*Are you getting enough to eat?* Nine out of ten people on this plan actually say they are now getting too much food (a strange complaint from someone on a diet!). They are afraid that they are eating enough to cancel out their weight loss altogether. Or they would like to eat less so that they can lose weight even faster. But *this will not happen.* Please eat all the food on the menu for Week Three. You won't lose more weight, or lose weight faster, by eliminating the fruit exchanges from your diet. You are exercising and burning calories at a good rate, and you need all of the food this diet prescribes.

Just try to accustom yourself to feeling full without feeling guilty!

*Do you feel hungry a lot of the time?* It happens very rarely, but once in a while a patient will experience hunger for the first time when fruit is added to the diet. If this should happen to you, it means that your body burns sugar very quickly, which tends to overstimulate your pancreas. As a result, too much insulin is produced and it burns blood sugar way down. And when your blood sugar is low, you feel hungry. Try taking the fruit with your meals rather than as a snack. This will delay the rapid absorption of sugar into your system.

This reaction indicates that your system doesn't respond well to "quick sugar," the type of sugar in fruit. "Quick sugar" is so called because it is already broken down and therefore is absorbed into your system faster than more complex types of sugar. If you really feel markedly different than you did during previous weeks, and if taking the fruit with meals doesn't assuage your hunger, I would advise notifying your doctor. He can test you for hypoglycemia.

If you don't feel the situation is serious enough to warrant such action—that is, if you are only mildly hungry, and even that is improved by taking the fruit with meals—then I can only assure you that you will feel better when you are in better physical shape. When you have a strong and healthy body, you'll be far more capable of handling the foods that may cause you trouble at this stage.

I always advocate eating everything allowed by the diet. But if fruit really is making you hungry, you may either decrease your exchanges or leave them out altogether for a week or two. Then try adding one exchange per day and see how you feel; if the hunger pangs are gone, add the second daily exchange too. You are healthier now, and your body can handle the fruit.

*Are you having trouble sleeping?* In this third week of exercise patients often feel that their sleep is disturbed. Often the complaint goes like this: "Doctor, I went to bed at ten as usual but couldn't get to sleep until eleven-thirty. I woke up at five-thirty and lay awake until seven, when I usually get up. What's *wrong?*" *Nothing* is wrong —everything is getting *right*. If this seems to be happening to you, ask yourself a few questions. Were you actually tired when you went to bed, or did you climb into your pajamas out of habit? Even though you missed some sleep that night, did you feel fatigued the next day? Or were you surprised to find you felt refreshed and alert, even though you'd had much less sleep than usual? The reason for all this is simple: the fit person needs less sleep. What seems like disturbed sleep is really the first signs of a stronger heart, stronger lungs, and improved body chemistry.

❉        ❉        ❉

Right about now you're probably thinking crafty, sneaky thoughts. So far you've been losing weight quite successfully on the test diet. You've found out a little about how you respond to carbohydrates and quick sugar, and now you've discovered that you need less sleep. Everything about the plan is great—except the exercise. You've been humoring me so far, but now in Week Three I'm putting you on the honor system and expecting you to exercise *and* figure out your own goals. It's just getting too complicated, so you're figuring you'll stick with the diet, but drop the exercise.

DON'T DO IT.

If you are reading this book straight through, you should remember why physical conditioning is essential to your success. But those of you who are reading week by week may have lost sight of our original goals and become discouraged with all the work you're doing. You've forgotten the message of the opening chapters: *Diet alone will never work.*

Consider Weight Watchers, reputed to be the most successful of all diet programs. Impressed by this organization's reputation, I decided to find out in person what they had to offer. I wasn't heavy enough to make the grade, though, so at the weighing-in I loaded my pockets with a hundred dollars' worth of quarters. Once admitted to the meetings, I found their outlook positive and enthusiastic. People were encouraged and applauded for any weight loss, and no one was ever chastised or humiliated

135

for gaining. Unfortunately, the Weight Watchers approach is unsatisfactory in two ways. First, at all the franchises I visited, the lecturers seemed ill-equipped to handle specific questions about nutrition. But what I feel is really tragic about WW is their determination to talk people out of exercise, using the old argument that exercise burns few calories while increasing one's appetite enormously.

My doubts about Weight Watchers were confirmed when we opened our clinic—and several of our first patients were Weight Watchers lecturers. These people's jobs depended on keeping their weight down, yet those pounds kept creeping back. On the Weight Watchers diet they lost, gained, lost a little, gained some, and on and on. . . .

If WW is off-base, you may be asking, why do so many people listen? WW has put its corporate finger on the perfect success formula: their philosophy appeals to those many fat people who are guided by inertia, to those who hate exercise to the point that getting up from the couch to change the TV channel is too much. You don't have to sweat, WW tells the fat one. —Good! says the fat person, that's just what I wanted to hear! —You don't even have to get out of your easy chair. —Good again! Without even changing my habits or way of life, I can become thin and beautiful. Terrific!

All Weight Watchers asks in return is that you diet —every day, every year—for the rest of your life. If you think that's easy—or even viable—ask the WW lecturers who came to my clinic to save their jobs.

The struggle does *not* have to go on and on like that. I'm constantly receiving letters from former patients attesting to the good effects exercise has had on their lives. One woman wrote me that she'd just returned from a Caribbean vacation where she ate lobster and conch and pompano and sipped banana daiquiris all day. She also ran on the beach every morning. When she returned home she weighed herself, expecting the worst. But *she hadn't gained one pound.*

This will happen to you too. The trouble is, we haven't come far enough yet for you to begin to feel the benefits of exercise. You've had eighteen activity sessions, enough to give you a sore muscle or two, but not enough to reveal a sleek and beautiful body. You *are* benefiting from all your work, but the results are not yet showing. As you come closer and closer to minimal physical fitness, your entire cardiovascular system is being strengthened. You have lost a lot of fat, and even more important, you are replacing that fat with lean body mass, so you're burning more calories per day than you ever did before. You are on the brink of seeing changes in your body and, just as wonderful, experiencing the new surge of energy I promised you as the reward of physical activity. You *will* look and feel terrific very, very soon. I guarantee it. So please, *stick with it!*

# Week Four

## WEEK FOUR DIET

This week's diet will consist of all the foods you've had in the previous two weeks, plus seven vegetable B exchanges per week. Again, you will learn about vegetable B's through problems on the following pages. They will teach you what you will need to know to integrate these new exchanges into your diet.

Respond to all questions and do not uncover the printed answer until you have formulated your own response.

    1.  Before we look at what is different about your diet for the

49
unlimited

fourth week, let's review what
we've learned in previous sections.
This diet plan allows you _____
meat exchanges a week and (*limited/unlimited*) amounts of vegetable A's as long as they are raw.

cooked

2. Your intake of vegetable A's
is limited only when you choose to
eat them (*raw/cooked*).

one

3. If you eat your vegetable A's
cooked, your intake is limited to
_____ cup per meal per day.

14

4. In addition to the meat exchanges and vegetable A's, you
may also eat 2 fruit exchanges
daily, or _____ fruit exchanges
weekly.

49

5. How many meat exchanges are
you allowed weekly on this diet?
Circle one:

39      16      49      14

6. On the vegetable B list, one
vegetable exchange contains 2

139

grams of protein and 7 grams of carbohydrate. Write the number of grams of carbohydrate and protein contained in one vegetable B exchange in the space provided below.

2

_____ grams protein in one vegetable B exchange.

7

_____ grams carbohydrate in one B exchange.

two
seven

7. There are t_____ grams of protein and se_____ grams of carbohydrate in one vegetable B exchange.

8. Circle the number of grams of protein contained in one vegetable B exchange.

2

6      0      2      1

9. Circle the number of grams of carbohydrate contained in one vegetable B exchange.

7

4      7      3      5

10. Since there are _____ grams of carbohydrate and _____ grams

140

$4 \times 7 = 28$
$4 \times 2 = \underline{\phantom{0}8}$
$\phantom{4 \times 2 = }36$

of protein in one exchange of vegetable B, and since each gram of protein and each gram of carbohydrate contains 4 calories, there must be a total of _____ calories in one vegetable B exchange.

11.   ½ cup of beets and ½ cup of carrots both contain 7 grams of carbohydrate and 2 grams of protein; ½ cup of beets and ½ cup of carrots, then, are both equal to _____ exchange on the vegetable B list.

one

12.   Since ½ cup of beets and ½ cup of carrots are both equal to one vegetable B exchange, if you wanted to do so, could you eat ½ cup of carrots instead of ½ cup of beets?

YES                                    YES        NO

Following is a list of the vegetables included in the vegetable B group, with the amounts necessary to equal one exchange. You will have to refer back to this list in answering the next questions.

## VEGETABLE B EXCHANGE EQUIVALENTS
### Each Item Equals One Vegetable B Exchange

| | |
|---|---|
| Beets | ½ cup |
| Carrots | ½ cup |
| Onions | ½ cup |
| Peas, green | ½ cup |
| Pumpkin | ½ cup |
| Rutabaga | ½ cup |
| Squash, winter | ½ cup |
| Turnips | ½ cup |

Now that you have two lists of vegetables to compare, you may notice that summer squash is on the unlimited vegetable A list, while winter squash is a vegetable B. Please remember that these food groups are based on the amount of proteins, carbohydrates, and fats each contains. Winter squash is much higher in carbohydrates than summer squash, so it is on the B list. Corn, which is missing from *both* lists, is so high in carbohydrates that it qualifies for the bread group (Week Seven).

Eat *only* the vegetables on the A and B lists. Some of your favorites, like corn, will be added to your diet later. Others you will be able to eat only *after* the forty-nine days.

1. Here is a list of vegetables. Check those that are included on the vegetable B list:

Beets
Pumpkin


Turnips

☐  Beets
☐  Pumpkin
☐  Potatoes
☐  Asparagus
☐  Turnips

½

2.  All the vegetables on the vegetable B list are equal to one exchange when used in amounts of _____ cup.

1

3.  This diet allows 7 exchanges of vegetable B's weekly. If you wanted to eat an equal number of vegetable B exchanges each day of the week, you would eat _____ exchange(s) a day.

4.  Write the number of exchanges each food is worth. Pay close attention to the amounts:

2

1 cup beets      = _____
            vegetable B exchange(s)

1

½ cup green peas = _____
            vegetable B exchange(s)

4

2 cups carrots   = _____
            vegetable B exchange(s)

143

5. Examine the following list to determine whether it is equal to 7 exchanges (the number of exchanges allowed weekly):

1 cup green peas
1 cup carrots
1½ cups pumpkin

a. YES                      a. YES      b. NO

6. Circle the number of vegetable exchanges you are allowed weekly:

7                      6    4    9    7

7. For our purposes, the vegetable B list differs from the vegetable A list in the amounts that you are allowed. You may have unlimited amounts of vegetable A's so long as you eat them uncooked, but you must limit your vegetable B's to
7       _____ exchanges a week, no matter how you prepare them.

You now know all you need to know in order to integrate the vegetable B exchanges into your diet. On the following page is a tally sheet for recording the amounts of meat, cooked vegetable A, fruit, and vegetable B exchanges you will eat in the coming week.

The total grams of carbohydrates, proteins, and fats per exchange this week are (per day):

|  | Carbohydrates | Proteins | Fats |
|---|---|---|---|
| Meat (7 per day) | 0 | 49 | 35 |
| Vegetable A's | 0 | 0 | 0 |
| Fruit (2 per day) | 20 | 0 | 0 |
| Vegetable B's (1 per day) | 7 | 2 | 0 |
| TOTAL GRAMS: | 27 | 51 | 35 |
| TOTAL CALORIES: | 108 | 204 | 315 = 627 per day |

Record the number of meat exchanges that you have for each meal or snack. You have a total of 49 exchanges for the week, so 7 per day is the proper average.

### MEAT EXCHANGES

| 1st Day | 2nd Day | 3rd Day | 4th Day | 5th Day | 6th Day | 7th Day |
|---|---|---|---|---|---|---|
|  |  |  |  |  |  |  |
|  |  |  |  |  |  |  |
|  |  |  |  |  |  |  |
|  |  |  |  |  |  |  |
|  |  |  |  |  |  |  |
|  |  |  |  |  |  |  |

TOTALS

145

Record the number of 1-cup portions of cooked vegetable A's that you have each day. You may eat unlimited amounts of raw vegetable A's, but you are limited to 1 cup per meal or 3 cups per day of cooked vegetable A's.

---

COOKED VEGETABLE A EXCHANGES

---

*1st Day  2nd Day  3rd Day  4th Day  5th Day  6th Day  7th Day*

---

TOTALS

---

Record the number of fruit exchanges that you have at each meal or snack. Remember that you are allowed to have 14 fruit exchanges per week, so try to keep the number of fruit exchanges you eat daily as close to 2 as possible to avoid having to do without fruit on the last day of Week Four.

---

FRUIT EXCHANGES

---

*1st Day  2nd Day  3rd Day  4th Day  5th Day  6th Day  7th Day*

---

TOTALS

---

146

Record the number of vegetable B exchanges that you have with each meal. You are allowed 7 vegetable B exchanges per week, or 1 per day.

VEGETABLE B EXCHANGES

*1st Day  2nd Day  3rd Day  4th Day  5th Day  6th Day  7th Day*

TOTALS

## WEEK FOUR EXERCISE

According to the guidelines charted on page 120, these are the goals for Week Four:

BIKERS:     3½ miles in 14 minutes
WALKERS:   2½ miles in 37½ minutes

However, as you know from our Week Three discussion of exercise, there is every possibility that those goals are not your goals.

If you achieved the Week Two goal by the end of Week Two or shortly thereafter, you are probably ahead of the Week Four guideline by now. If so, don't cheat and give yourself an easy week by working on a goal you've already surpassed. Continue pushing yourself to do as much as you *safely* can every day.

147

If the Week Four guideline is still beyond you, don't feel that you are falling behind. As I mentioned in Week Three, the walkers' goal is a tough one, and it will normally take some extra time. After all, it's taken you a long time to get out of condition, so it's only natural for your body to need a bit more time to get back *into* shape. Above all, don't get frantic and start overtaxing yourself. Continue exercising as hard as you safely can, and continue testing yourself to see if you can safely improve your distance. But keep a careful finger on your pulse every time you exercise, and test yourself. Once you pass a certain stage in your reconditioning, your progress will be faster. There is no point in rushing things now.

Not all of you will be far beyond or far below the demands of the Week Four guideline. Perhaps you've found you can bike 3½ miles, but it takes 15 minutes instead of 14. Or you can walk 2½ miles, but you require 40 minutes instead of 37½. That's fine: this week work at cutting down your time gradually. If you meet the Week Four goal after only a couple of days, continue with that distance for a few more days, then test yourself on the next guideline.

REMEMBER:

Warm up and cool down after every exercise period.

Be demanding of yourself, but sensible.

Check your pulse daily to be sure you're staying within your training range.

## WEEK FOUR PROBLEMS

We see two major problems during Week Four—guilt about eating too much, and the plateau. These problems will continue to be with some of us for the remaining weeks of the plan.

By now you are eating fairly large quantities of food. You feel full after every meal and this feeling elicits the old guilts you've always associated with eating binges.

You may be looking at your plate and thinking that this plan, this book, and its author are surely playing some sort of cruel joke on you. There is just too much food there. And it tastes too good.

You want to cut back, to return to your old method of starvation (alternating with binges). Fat people starve without much trouble, so, to make sure that you do lose weight, you're fully prepared to go hungry for a few more weeks.

But I *want* you to feel full. You need to eat all the nourishing foods on this plan even though you have none of the nagging appetite problems you experienced with past diets.

I strongly encourage you to eat all of your food exchanges.

When you do, your daily diet in Week Four still totals less than 700 calories!

You are increasing your physical activity, so that, if you are consuming only 700 calories per day, you will ex-

149

perience very satisfying weight losses. You will not be hungry and yet you will continue to lose weight and improve your figure.

By Week Four, you are eating meat, two groups of vegetables, and fruit. You've learned how your body reacts to these foods and you're experiencing gratifying losses. This positive feedback, coupled with a lack of hunger, means that you will succeed. The physical activity is gradually allowing you to eat more and more, your body is changing, you're looking better, and a meal is not an agonizing wrestling match between your appetite and your willpower. You will succeed.

The plateau is the most difficult and dangerous problem for any dieter. Everyone at some time or other reaches a "plateau," a period when, despite all your good work, you lose practically nothing. The scale stares back at you with the same numbers day after discouraging day.

A plateau due to fat loss alone can last for about two weeks. A plateau due to better conditioning is rarely shorter than three weeks, but could conceivably last as long as seven weeks. (I have seen this only two or three times in my experience, but it *is* a possibility.)

During this time you will feel most discouraged. It is terribly depressing, after making the psychological effort four weeks ago to go on a diet, and after faithfully observing all the rules, to see a stalled scale, the indicator reading back the same poundage every day.

Try not to give the scale so much power over your spirits. *If you are following this plan faithfully, you are losing weight, even though your scale does not show it.* Fat *is* being burned off your body because you aren't feeding yourself enough calories to maintain the fat and because your physical activity demands more and more calories.

So stay with the plan, even in this discouraging time.

Notice your clothes. Are they looser around the waist? Have they been looser almost every morning since you began on the plan? Are you buckling your belt a notch or more tighter?

Doesn't this tell you something about your progress? Are you beginning to believe me when I tell you not to pay attention to your scale?

Use your scale, but don't let it use you. When it shows a weight loss, that's good. When it doesn't, that doesn't mean you haven't lost fat. You have.

Plateaus are rough. It takes time for your body to adjust to its new, healthier state. Give yourself the time your body needs by continuing with this plan.

When you break through the plateau, it will be the greatest dieting experience of your life. In a single week, you will suddenly lose up to 10 pounds, all the pounds you couldn't seem to lose in the previous weeks. You will have a joyous experience because your faith in your own ability to succeed has been rewarded.

Suddenly, within the space of a single week, you will

begin adjusting your image of yourself. You will begin to see yourself as a slimmer person. You will look forward to living every day fully and happily. These rewards are well worth a few more days' patience right now.

If your weight loss has suddenly halted, there is one other possible explanation. The vegetable B group that you added this week contains seven grams of carbohydrates per exchange, only a few grams less than the carbohydrates in one fruit exchange. If you are a person who is particularly sensitive to carbohydrates, maybe the vegetable B's have stopped your weight loss. To find out, drop these exchanges from your diet for three days. If you go back to losing weight within three days, it means you must be particularly careful about other carbohydrate-containing food groups, especially milk in Week Six and bread in Week Seven. If after three days without vegetable B's you are still not losing weight, you *are* on a plateau and may as well continue eating vegetable B's while your body works it through.

Even if vegetable B's do seem to be the source of your problem, eliminate them for only two weeks. Then try to reintroduce them into your diet. Your body is changing every day, and within two weeks your body chemistry may have normalized sufficiently for you to digest vegetable B's without causing abnormal weight gain.

Even if your weight loss has temporarily halted, you have reasons for feeling good during Week Four. You should be experiencing a sense of well-being, which results from your improved physical condition. You don't need as much sleep as you used to, and you have more energy during the day.

Your *real* body, dormant for so long, is beginning to come alive. If you've ever watched your dog chase a squirrel, I'm sure you'll agree that he looks much more beautiful with his whole body straining forward than when he's sacked out on your living-room floor, or staring lazily across the front lawn. The same goes for your own body.

Believe me, I have nothing against television; you can find me in front of one whenever there's a good ball game or movie on. But I don't think our bodies were intended to prop us up in front of a TV screen. Since I've become healthy, my whole attitude toward life has changed so drastically that I feel different even when I'm sitting quietly watching TV. I don't have to prop my legs up because they're tired and aching. I don't have to slouch down in my chair because it's easier to breathe that way. I don't have to hold my head up with one hand.

This new way of life will soon be yours, and this is the week that it's beginning. Now is the time to begin asking yourself: do I feel a little bit better about myself each day? If the answer is yes, perhaps you will face your daily activity period with a little more enthusiasm than you did the day before. The longer you diet, the hungrier you get, and the more unwilling you become to continue dieting. Exercise has just the opposite effect; it is self-reinforcing. The longer you exercise, the better you feel, and the more

153

you look forward to your exercise period. If you are beginning to feel that way now, you are only a few weeks away from becoming an exercise junkie. Congratulations! You are far along the road to being formerly fat.

Nice going.

# Week Five

## WEEK FIVE DIET

This week we will add a much-maligned but necessary food group, the fats. You probably think they are dangerous, but we are inserting them into your diet in a safe, limited way because, whether you know it or not, you need them.

To us, fat is the enemy. Putting a gram of fat into our mouths constitutes an act of self-sabotage, or maybe even madness. Primitive man, of course, was happy to eat all the fats he could get—they provided calories that he could store for less prosperous times. But even though we now worry more about avoiding calories than acquiring them, fats are still necessary. Nutritionally, they supply what are called "essential fatty acids," and fat soluble vitamins. No dieter should ever try to eliminate fat entirely. Important as these fatty acids are, however, you don't need fat exchanges to get them—they can be provided indirectly in the forty-nine meat exchanges you are eating every week.

For the purposes of this diet, fats are being added for two other reasons. Though the kinds and quantities of food we're adding here won't exactly constitute a feast, they will return to your diet some of the good tastes you've missed in the last four weeks. Fats are also useful to the dieter because their satiety value is high. Eating a few fats will leave you satisfied enough to resist a starch or carbohydrate binge.

So dismiss your doubts about fats and go on to the following set of questions, remembering to cover the printed answers until you have formulated your own response.

$9 \times 5 = 45$

1. One fat exchange contains 5 grams of fat. One gram of fat contains 9 calories. Thus one fat exchange contains _____ calories.

five

2. There are fi_____ grams of fat in every fat exchange.

3. You are allowed 14 fat exchanges weekly. If you wanted to

2

have an equal number of fat exchanges for each day of the coming week, you would have _____ fat exchanges daily.

Circle the number of fat exchanges that you may have each *week* on this diet.

14

9    7    14    12

Here is a list of the foods that equal one fat exchange when used in the amounts indicated. You will have to refer back to this list in formulating your answers to the next few questions.

---

### FAT EXCHANGE EQUIVALENTS

*Each Item Equals One Exchange*

| | |
|---|---|
| Avocado (4″ diameter) | ⅛ |
| Bacon, crisp | 1 slice |
| Butter or Margarine | 1 teaspoon |
| Cream Cheese | 1 tablespoon |
| Cream, heavy | 1 tablespoon |
| Cream, light | 2 tablespoons |
| Mayonnaise | 1 teaspoon |
| Nondietetic salad dressing | 1 tablespoon |
| Nuts | 6 small |
| Oil or cooking fat | 1 teaspoon |
| Olives | 5 small |

---

1.   Here is a list of foods, some of which are included on the fat ex-

change list and some of which are not. Check the foods that are *not* included on the fat exchange list:

Milk

Potatoes

Potato chips
Pork chops

Cottage cheese

☐ Cream, light
☐ Milk
☐ Nuts
☐ Potatoes
☐ Bacon
☐ Potato chips
☐ Pork chops
☐ Cream cheese
☐ Cottage cheese
☐ French dressing

2. How many fat exchanges are contained in the foods listed next? Pay close attention to quantities:

2

1

1

2 teaspoons margarine =
_____ fat exchange(s)
1 teaspoon mayonnaise =
_____ fat exchange(s)
⅛ small avocado =
_____ fat exchange(s)

3. You are allowed 14 fat exchanges weekly. Does this list add up to 14 exchanges?
4 teaspoons butter

10 tablespoons light cream
5 slices crisp bacon

YES                    YES          NO

Fat exchanges, as you have seen, are fairly easy to understand. All you need to remember is that you are allowed 14 fat exchanges each week. Be sure to refer to your Fat Exchange Equivalents list to see that you are using the proper amounts.

Record the number of meat exchanges that you eat each day.

Stay as close to 7 meat exchanges daily as possible.

## MEAT EXCHANGES

| 1st Day | 2nd Day | 3rd Day | 4th Day | 5th Day | 6th Day | 7th Day |
|---------|---------|---------|---------|---------|---------|---------|
|         |         |         |         |         |         |         |
|         |         |         |         |         |         |         |
|         |         |         |         |         |         |         |
|         |         |         |         |         |         |         |
|         |         |         |         |         |         |         |
|         |         |         |         |         |         |         |

TOTALS

Record the number of cooked vegetable A's that you eat each day. You are allowed ½ cup cooked vegetable A's per meal per day.

### COOKED VEGETABLE A EXCHANGES

| 1st Day | 2nd Day | 3rd Day | 4th Day | 5th Day | 6th Day | 7th Day |
| --- | --- | --- | --- | --- | --- | --- |

TOTALS

Record the number of fruit exchanges that you have each day. You are allowed 14 fruit exchanges; try to use 2 exchanges a day.

### FRUIT EXCHANGES

| 1st Day | 2nd Day | 3rd Day | 4th Day | 5th Day | 6th Day | 7th Day |
| --- | --- | --- | --- | --- | --- | --- |

TOTALS

Record the number of vegetable B exchanges that you eat each day. You are allowed a total of 7 vegetable B exchanges a week; try to use 1 exchange each day.

### VEGETABLE B EXCHANGES

| 1st Day | 2nd Day | 3rd Day | 4th Day | 5th Day | 6th Day | 7th Day |
| --- | --- | --- | --- | --- | --- | --- |

TOTALS

Record the number of fat exchanges that you eat each day. You are allowed a total of 14 fat exchanges for the entire week; try to use 2 exchanges each day.

## FAT EXCHANGES

| | 1st Day | 2nd Day | 3rd Day | 4th Day | 5th Day | 6th Day | 7th Day |
|---|---|---|---|---|---|---|---|
| | | | | | | | |
| | | | | | | | |
| TOTALS | | | | | | | |
| | | | | | | | |

The total number of grams per exchange available to you this week are (per day):

| | Carbohydrates | Proteins | Fats |
|---|---|---|---|
| Meat (7 per day) | 0 | 49 | 35 |
| Vegetable A's | 0 | 0 | 0 |
| Fruit (2 per day) | 20 | 0 | 0 |
| Vegetable B's (1 per day) | 7 | 2 | 0 |
| Fat (2 per day) | 0 | 0 | 10 |
| TOTAL GRAMS: | 27 | 51 | 45 |
| TOTAL CALORIES: | 108 | 204 | 405 = 717 per day |

161

## WEEK FIVE EXERCISE

According to the chart on page 120, these are the guidelines for Week Five:

BIKERS:        4 miles in 16 minutes
WALKERS:     3 miles in 45 minutes

This week some of you who have been progressing slowly will begin to catch up. For you this week is very important, since it signals a turning point in your progress toward fitness. After this week your exercise periods will not be so laborious. They will still require a lot of effort, but you will feel your body responding to the challenge, and your confidence in your own ability will make the task easier.

Some of you will find that these goals reflect your own goals fairly accurately. You are progressing at a normal pace, and you should feel very satisfied: success will be yours, probably in Week Seven or shortly thereafter. But now is not the time to relax. Once you've achieved the Week Five goal, don't keep putting off the test for Week Six. You'll be able to handle it very soon.

Have you already reached the Week Seven goal? Congratulations. No more tests, no more pulse readings— but you *must* continue your daily activity periods. The forty-nine days are still not over; you must continue the test diet, as well as your exercise, until the end of the seventh week. At that point, when many others have joined you in achieving the Week Seven goal and everyone is at least within striking distance of it, we will discuss where to go from there with your diet and exercise. Meanwhile: bravo. If you continue to bike 6 miles in 24 minutes or walk 4 miles in 60 minutes *every day,* you will continue to lose until you have reached your ideal weight. And you will never be fat again.

## WEEK FIVE PROBLEMS

You've stuck out this plan for thirty-five days, and now the worst is behind you. I'm sure you've been amazed by how far you've progressed. For those of you whose weight loss has been slowed or stopped by a plateau, this week you will definitely begin to lose your water weight, and the remaining weeks will be downhill. Let me qualify all these promises and guarantees: I naturally assume you haven't been cheating! You've exercised diligently and stuck to the diet. I wish you could lose weight just by reading, but no one can write *that* persuasively.

This is the time when the real benefits of the plan begin to manifest themselves in every case. Many people began to feel good earlier than this week, but by now almost all of you should feel markedly better, even though you haven't yet lost all you want to.

Still, in the fifth week, I do encounter exceptional patients who continue to complain of fatigue, and feel as tired as they did before they began. A good example is Eleanor, a thirty-eight-year-old housewife and mother of three. Despite her excellent progress in the physical activity program, she still felt tired in Week Five. In the group I was treating at the time she was the only patient who didn't feel great, so I advised her to go to her family doctor for a checkup. I was astonished when she reported back to me that she had a hypothyroid condition. I say "astonished" because this same family doctor had tested Eleanor *five times* previously, but her condition had been consistently disguised by her lack of fitness. Once she began to take medication for the thyroid condition, her weight loss accelerated, her spirits soared, and she had all the energy that the rest of my Week Five patients did.

I must stress that you cannot make a self-diagnosis. If you're still feeling fatigued at this point, don't nod your head and say, "Aah, that's it—thyroid." See your doctor for a thorough checkup; there are many possibilities when it comes to diagnosing fatigue, so investigate as soon as possible so you can get back on the program.

Did you discover that you stopped losing weight this week? Like continued fatigue, this problem is very rare during Week Five, but occasionally it occurs. If you are one of the unlucky few, try eating only one fat exchange per day for the rest of the week. If weight loss does not resume, then your fat exchanges are the culprit and you should eliminate them from your diet for two weeks. Be very watchful during Week Six. Milk will be added to your diet that week, and you are particularly sensitive to all fats, even those in whole milk.

Do not eliminate fats entirely unless you *have* to, and don't be afraid you will have to stay away from fats forever. Like fruit, vegetable B's, and any other food that may have given you trouble earlier in the test diet, fats will eventually be digested normally and easily when you reach fitness and normalize your body chemistry.

Are you remembering to eat slowly? When I was in Week Five, my wife timed a meal I had on an airplane. I was horrified when she told me I'd consumed salad, main course, and tea in six minutes flat! Because of my greediness, I had to sit there and feel hungry for ten minutes after the meal, whereas if I had taken thirty minutes to eat, I would have felt fuller. Thereafter I concentrated on slowing down my meals, and it really does work: less tastes like more when you eat slowly.

Now that you have much more food in your daily diet, you might find it helpful to write down everything you eat. It was very interesting and enlightening for both me and my patients when I asked them to do this at the clinic. Everyone wrote very quickly. One, two, three, done. Then I asked one woman how she had spent her day. Shopping, this, that, PTA meeting.

"Did they serve cookies and coffee at the PTA?" I asked.

"Sure they did," she said.

"I see from your list that you didn't have any cookies there, Lynn. That was very good. . . ."

"Oh . . . wait . . . I, um, forgot. I *did* have a couple of little ones."

Not that Lynn was singled out for embarrassment; going around the group one by one, I found that almost everybody was able to add at least one delightful nibble they'd had during the day, something so tiny—and so caloric—it had conveniently slipped from memory.

Many fat people are inveterate tasters; while preparing a meal, they take a sip of this and an itsy-bitsy bite of that, just to make sure everything's right. By the time the meal hits the table, you may have eaten as much in the kitchen as you will in the dining room! So don't let yourself put anything over on yourself. Keep careful record of everything that goes into your mouth. The skinny you has to fight the fathead you the whole way.

Even though you have fat exchanges in your diet now, you can save them for good things to eat if you use Teflon cookware. That way you won't need to use precious exchanges for cooking oil. Spray-on vegetable coatings are also free of fats, so you may use them too.

Unless you object to margarine, very strongly, use it instead of butter. And read margarine labels carefully.

Some of those that advertise "more butter flavor" actually do contain butter.

Continue using diet salad dressing so that you can use your fat exchanges on snacks. Don't deny yourself the treats these fat exchanges allow. If you're still not convinced that you can eat limited amounts of fat safely, think back on Week Two. Meat has five grams of fat per exchange, which is exactly the amount of fat in one fat exchange. And in the last five weeks you lost a lot of weight while eating many, many meat exchanges. So go ahead and treat yourself. Besides being delicious, a bowl of blueberries and heavy cream (no sugar yet, please!) can convince you much more graphically than I ever could that you *are* becoming a normal, slim, healthy person who can eat some of the foods you love without gaining weight.

# Week Six

## WEEK SIX DIET

This week we will add the milk exchanges to your diet. You will continue to eat all the foods you ate during Week Two through Week Five, plus seven milk exchanges per week, or an average of one per day.

Following is a set of questions about the milk exchanges. Remember to respond to all the questions and avoid consulting the printed answers before you have given your own responses.

1. One milk exchange contains 12 grams of carbohydrate, 8 grams of protein, and 10 grams of fat. Fill

in the numbers of grams of the three basic foodstuffs contained in one milk exchange:

12 ———— grams carbohydrate in 1 milk exchange.

8 ———— grams protein in 1 milk exchange.

10 ———— grams fat in 1 milk exchange.

2. One gram of carbohydrate contains 4 calories. Since there are 12 grams of carbohydrate in one milk exchange, the carbohydrate content of one milk exchange provides

48 ———— calories.

3. How many grams of carbohydrate are contained in one milk exchange? Circle one:

12        6     9     12     16

4. One gram of fat contains 9 calories. There are 10 grams of fat in one milk exchange; therefore the fat content in a milk exchange provides

90 vides ———— calories.

169

5. Circle the number of grams of fat contained in one milk exchange:

10

      6      4      10      20

6. One gram of protein contains 4 calories. There are 8 grams of protein in one milk exchange and therefore there are _____ calories provided by the protein content of one milk exchange.

32

7. Circle the number of grams of protein contained in one milk exchange:

8

      1      6      8      10

8. Match the foodstuff listed here with the number of *grams* of that foodstuff contained in one milk exchange.

b. 12       Carbohydrates _____ a. 6
c. 8        Proteins     _____ b. 12
d. 10      Fats         _____ c. 8
                                   d. 10

9. One cup of whole milk and one cup of buttermilk both con-

exchange

tain 12 grams of carbohydrate, 8 grams of protein and 10 grams of fat. One cup of each of these foods is equal to one milk _____.

exchange

10. Any milk _____ may be taken in place of any other milk

exchange

_____.

Here is a list of milk products in amounts equal to one milk exchange. You will have to refer back to this list in formulating your answers to the next few problems.

---

### MILK EXCHANGE EQUIVALENTS

*Each Item Equals One Exchange*

| | |
|---|---|
| Whole milk (plain or homogenized) | 1 cup |
| *Skim milk | 1 cup |
| Evaporated milk | ½ cup |
| Powdered whole milk | ¼ cup |
| Powdered skim milk (non-fat dried milk) | ¼ cup |
| Buttermilk (made from whole milk) | 1 cup |
| *Buttermilk (made from skim milk) | 1 cup |

---

\* *Skim milk and skim buttermilk contain less fat than whole-milk products, but their sugar and protein content are the same. Consider them as equal for the purposes of the milk exchange, but see questions 1 to 5 on pages 174-175.*

You may be disappointed not to find ice cream on the milk list. But if you think about it, ice cream is much sweeter (that is, higher in sugar content) than these foods. You *will* find ice cream on the bread list, in Week Seven.

1. Place a check in the square next to the foods listed here that are *not* included on the milk exchange list.

| | |
|---|---|
| | ☐ Buttermilk |
| Cream, light | ☐ Cream, light |
| | ☐ Powdered whole milk |
| Cheese | ☐ Cheese |
| | ☐ Evaporated milk |
| Ice cream | ☐ Ice cream |

2. Write the amounts necessary to make each of the foods listed below equal to one milk exchange.

| | | |
|---|---|---|
| 1 cup | Buttermilk | _____ |
| ¼ cup | Powdered skim milk | _____ |
| 1 cup | Skim milk | _____ |
| ½ cup | Evaporated milk | _____ |

3. Suppose you wanted to use only one milk exchange on a given day and you have already drunk ½ cup of whole milk at breakfast.

How much buttermilk could you drink without exceeding your one milk exchange limitation? Circle one:

½ cup

¾ cup      1 cup

½ cup      ⅔ cup

4. If you wanted to use two exchanges of powdered milk in a recipe, how much would you measure out? _____ powdered milk.

½ cup

5. This diet allows you 7 milk exchanges weekly. If you wanted to have an equal number of milk exchanges each day, you would use _____ milk exchange(s) daily.

1

6. One cup of whole milk equals one milk exchange. If you were to drink 7 cups of milk in a week, would you be adhering to your limitation for milk exchanges?

YES

YES      NO

7. Circle the number of milk exchanges allowed weekly on this diet:

7

5     3     7     9

You are allowed 7 milk exchanges a week on this diet. However, if you elect to use only skim milk products to satisfy your milk exchange allotment, you may also have an extra 14 fat exchanges a week.

Study the following information.
One milk exchange contains:
12 grams carbohydrate
8 grams protein
*10 grams fat*

One fat exchange contains:
*5 grams fat*

1. From the information you just read, you can see that 1 milk exchange contains:

a. The same number of grams of fat as *1 fat exchange*.

b. Same as 2 fat exchanges

b. The same number of grams of fat as *2 fat exchanges*.

2. One milk exchange contains 10 grams of fat. Two fat exchanges also contain _____ grams of fat.

10

That is why you are allowed to eat

2

an extra _____ fat exchanges every time you use skim milk prod-

174

ucts, since skim milk products contain no fats.

3.  I used skim milk for my milk exchange on Monday and whole milk for my milk exchange on Tuesday. I can have two extra fat exchanges on:

a. Monday

    a.  Monday.
    b.  Neither day.
    c.  Monday and Tuesday.

4.  For every day that you use skim milk products for your milk exchange you may have an extra _____ fat exchanges. Circle the number of extra fat exchanges you would be allowed if you used skim milk products for all your weekly milk exchanges.

2

14

    7     12     11     14

7

skim
2

5.  You are allowed _____ milk exchanges a week. Every time you use _____ milk products you may also have an extra _____ fat exchanges.

175

You now know all you need to know in order to integrate your daily and weekly allotments of milk exchanges into your diet. On this and the following pages are tally sheets for recording the numbers of exchanges you will be eating during the next week. Be sure that you record everything you eat on the tally sheets because, given the variety and amounts of food you are now eating, you may easily forget how many exchanges you have left, and eat too much or too little.

You have 49 meat exchanges for the week. Stay as close to 7 meat exchanges daily as possible.

## MEAT EXCHANGES

| 1st Day | 2nd Day | 3rd Day | 4th Day | 5th Day | 6th Day | 7th Day |
|---------|---------|---------|---------|---------|---------|---------|
| | | | | | | |
| | | | | | | |
| | | | | | | |
| | | | | | | |
| | | | | | | |
| | | | | | | |
| TOTALS | | | | | | |
| | | | | | | |

You are allowed ½ cup cooked vegetable A's per meal per day.

## COOKED VEGETABLE A EXCHANGES

*1st Day  2nd Day  3rd Day  4th Day  5th Day  6th Day  7th Day*

TOTALS

You are allowed a total of 14 fruit exchanges. Stay as close to 2 exchanges a day as possible.

## FRUIT EXCHANGES

*1st Day  2nd Day  3rd Day  4th Day  5th Day  6th Day  7th Day*

TOTALS

You are allowed a total of 7 vegetable B exchanges a week, so keep the amounts you eat as close to 1 exchange daily as possible.

## VEGETABLE B EXCHANGES

*1st Day  2nd Day  3rd Day  4th Day  5th Day  6th Day  7th Day*

TOTALS

177

You are allowed a total of 14 fat exchanges for the entire week, so keep your daily consumption as close to 2 exchanges as possible.

---

### FAT EXCHANGES

| 1st Day | 2nd Day | 3rd Day | 4th Day | 5th Day | 6th Day | 7th Day |
|---------|---------|---------|---------|---------|---------|---------|

TOTALS

You are allowed a total of 7 milk exchanges weekly, so keep your daily consumption as close to 1 exchange as possible. Total each day as you go along.

---

### MILK EXCHANGES

| 1st Day | 2nd Day | 3rd Day | 4th Day | 5th Day | 6th Day | 7th Day |
|---------|---------|---------|---------|---------|---------|---------|

TOTALS

The total number of grams of carbohydrates, proteins, and fats per exchange eaten this week are (per day):

|  | Carbohydrates | Proteins | Fats |
|---|---|---|---|
| Meat (7 per day) | 0 | 49 | 35 |
| Vegetable A's | 0 | 0 | 0 |
| Fruit (2 per day) | 20 | 0 | 0 |
| Vegetable B's (1 per day) | 7 | 2 | 0 |
| Fat (2 per day) | 0 | 0 | 10 |
| Milk (1 per day) | 12 | 8 | 10 |
|  | — | — | — |
| TOTAL GRAMS: | 39 | 59 | 55 |
| TOTAL CALORIES: | 156 | 236 | 495 = 887 per day |

## WEEK SIX EXERCISE

The guidelines for Week Six are as follows:

BIKERS:      5 miles in 20 minutes
WALKERS:     3½ miles in 52½ minutes

By now you all know where you stand in relation to those general figures. If you've already achieved the Week Seven goal, continue exercising daily. You're probably feeling so good by now that you don't need any further encouragement. So let me give you a reminder instead: don't ever forget that you owe all your good feelings of health and energy to *exercise, not diet.* And although you may eventually go off the diet, when you have lost all the weight you want to lose, *you will never stop exercising, every day for the rest of your life.*

For those of you still moving along toward your ultimate goal—and that's most of you—I have a different reminder: *the duration and intensity of your exercise is vital.* Suppose you can now ride 7 miles on your bike instead of the 5 miles the plan calls for—but instead of 20 minutes it takes you an hour. I hope you're enjoying the ride, because the exercise is doing very little good. Sure, you're burning almost the same number of calories, whether you ride 5 miles in 20 minutes or 7 miles in an hour. But you are not building LBM; you are not strengthening your heart and lungs; and you are not normalizing your body chemistry.

The same goes for walkers. Maybe you've figured out that you walk 3 miles in the course of your usual eight-hour work day. But that walking has nothing to do with this plan. If you're not *also* doing your special 3½-mile walk in 52½ minutes, you're not getting anywhere. Even if you do lose 30 pounds or more in the seven weeks, there's no guarantee you'll keep those pounds off, because you haven't made the necessary changes in your body.

So don't lose sight of the purposes of this plan. Don't get sloppy now, just as we're coming into the home stretch. Continue exercising, even if you're still more than a week away from this week's goal. Soon you will be feeling so terrific that you'll be willing to carry on your exercise long after the forty-nine days have ended. I promise.

## WEEK SIX PROBLEMS

The ad says: "Everybody needs milk." I don't believe it. Another ad says: "Milk has something for everybody." I do believe *that*. Milk has saturated fats, which can lead to heart trouble. It has a lot of calcium, which may cause kidney stones in an adult past the growth years. It has lactose, a form of sugar that many black people cannot digest properly. For these people, milk means a stomachache.

We have a milk mania in this country and, as far as I'm concerned, there's no good reason for it. Nature designed milk for baby cows. Even adult cows don't drink the stuff, and there's no reason to think that milk ideally suits the nutritional needs of adult human beings.

Some nutritionists would argue that a diet without milk is deficient in calcium. I believe that, as an adult, you are obtaining sufficient quantities of calcium from the other foods you are eating.

So try your milk exchanges this week. But this is one food group that you may feel completely free to drop *after a one-week tryout*. (If your calcium intake worries you, each day take the lowest available dosage of an inexpensive calcium supplement pill.) Remember, milk has 170 calories per glass. If you don't really like its taste, but feel you deserve those calories as part of the diet, use it in cooking some dish you especially enjoy. Otherwise it's perfectly all right to pass it up entirely.

Did the milk exchanges you used this week cause abdominal cramps, gas, or increased hunger or thirst? If so, definitely drop the milk exchanges. Such symptoms indicate that your body does not process the lactose in milk efficiently.

You are reaching the end of the forty-nine-day plan. After one more week of exchange dieting, you will be free to eat whatever you want. And then all the old temptations will present themselves to you once again.

How will you react?

Now is a good time to ask yourself: Why do I eat? Fat people eat for so many reasons besides hunger—they eat out of loneliness, boredom, anxiety, and nervousness. They are often angry and jealous people who decide that they really *want* to be fat. Sometimes they convince themselves that they *need* the cloak of obesity—it excuses them from social and sexual competition, which they are certain they will lose.

If none of this applies to you, think about your own reasons for eating when you're not hungry. And once you've figured some of them out, dream up effective ways to combat your own psychology. If you are bored, for example, make an effort to fill your time with activity that you truly enjoy and find fulfilling. There are so many possibilities: studying guitar, sewing, knitting, volunteer work in local schools and hospitals, political campaign work, even yoga. Putting food in your mouth to fulfill other needs is just too easy. You have to make an effort to fill your life with things you enjoy—every day. And soon it will cease to be an effort.

By now you know that dieting alone won't solve your weight problems. Only a balanced diet and physical activity will. Yet new diet books are published every day telling you that you can glut yourself on certain foods and still lose weight. You can't—not safely, not permanently. I say you can eat all you want, once you are physically fit, and that is true. But you should still ask yourself why you would ever *want* to eat like a glutton.

A former patient wrote me that, having achieved maximal physical fitness, he could eat a pound of butter at one sitting with no weight gain. But, he complained, he always gained weight after eating a pound of candy. He wondered if I could explain why that was so. Instead of giving an answer, I asked him a question: Why eat a pound of either one? Who needs to eat a pound of butter?

So stop and think for a moment before you eat. That moment may save you an extra pound you'll have to work off later.

Are you continuing to lose weight steadily? If you are still on a plateau, you are no more than a few days away from the weight loss I have been predicting for you. You *are* losing fat, and the water and salt you are retaining will leave you any day now. I promise.

Maybe you hit a plateau two or three weeks ago and fought through it, but this week you've suddenly stopped losing inches or weight. You are most probably experiencing some of the symptoms I described earlier (abdominal pains, gas, hunger, thirst). You're having trouble digesting milk.

Give up the milk exchanges and increase your physical activity to two exercise periods a day. Double sessions are necessary *for just a few days*, to counteract the effects of the milk. Chances are very good that your ancestors had a great talent for storing calories efficiently—and you're the unhappy heir of that once-valuable ability. You need relatively few calories to maintain your body weight, and if you give up this plan you'll probably gain about 10 pounds a year until you weigh in at 200 or 300.

Stick with the plan. You are getting into shape slowly, but if you persist, you will *increase* you caloric need and thereby defeat your heredity. Now you know the cause of your obesity *and* the solution. So don't be depressed. For you, increased LBM is the only answer. All you have to do is keep *exercising*.

# Week Seven

## WEEK SEVEN DIET

This week we will encounter the most dangerous food group of all. But we're not going to worry about it. By now your body should be ready to handle bread with little trouble. And eating bread is the only way to find out for sure how you react to it.

Your diet will consist of all the exchanges you've had in the previous six weeks, plus *28 bread exchanges per week, plus 14 additional meat exchanges per week.*

Thus your diet for this week (and, as I will explain in the next chapter, for as long as you wish to remain on this plan) will consist of the following foods:

☐   63 meat exchanges
☐   unlimited uncooked vegetable A's
☐   7 vegetable B exchanges
☐   14 fruit exchanges
☐   7 milk exchanges
☐   28 bread exchanges

You have already learned all you need to know about meat exchanges (if you need a refresher, see page 84), so the only thing you'll have to remember about adding more meat exchanges to your diet is that you should try to keep the number of meat exchanges in your daily menu as close to 9 as possible (to equal a total of 63 meat exchanges per week).

Questions on the bread exchanges follow. Keep the printed answers covered until you have figured out your own responses.

1. One bread exchange contains 15 grams carbohydrate and 2 grams of protein. Fill in the number of grams of carbohydrate and protein contained in one bread exchange:

15        _____ grams carbohydrate in one bread exchange.

2         _____ grams protein in one bread exchange.

2. Carbohydrates and proteins both contain 4 calories to the gram.

15
2
$15 \times 4 = 60$
$2 \times 4 = +8$
_____
68

One bread exchange contains _____ grams of carbohydrates and _____ grams of protein, so there must be a total of _____ calories in one bread exchange.

3. Circle the number of grams of carbohydrate contained in one bread exchange:

15

6        12        15        9

4. Circle the number of grams of protein contained in one bread exchange.

2

3        6        7        2

5. One small potato and ½ cup cooked spaghetti both contain 2 grams of protein and 15 grams of carbohydrate. Each of these foods, then, equals one br_____ exchange.

bread

6. Since 1 small white potato and ½ cup of cooked spaghetti are both equal to one bread exchange, could

you eat a small white potato instead of ½ cup of cooked spaghetti?

YES                    YES        NO

7. This diet allows 28 bread exchanges weekly. If you wanted to eat an equal number of bread exchanges each day of the week, you

4        would eat _____ bread exchanges daily.

Here is the bread exchange list. In the amounts listed each item equals one bread exchange. Refer back to this list in answering the next few questions.

---

### BREAD EXCHANGE EQUIVALENTS
*Each Item Equals One Bread Exchange*

| | |
|---|---|
| Any kind of bread | 1 slice |
| Biscuit, roll, 2″ diameter | 1 |
| Muffin, 2″ diameter | 1 |
| Cereal, cooked | ½ cup |
| Cereal, dry | ¾ cup |
| Rice, grits, cooked | ½ cup |
| Spaghetti, cooked | ½ cup |
| Noodles or other pasta, cooked | ½ cup |
| Crackers, graham, 2½″ square | 5 |
| Oyster | 20 (½ cup) |
| Saltines, 2″ square | 5 |
| Soda, 2½″ square | 3 |

---

## BREAD EXCHANGE EQUIVALENTS *(cont'd)*
### *Each Item Equals One Bread Exchange*

| | |
|---|---|
| Round, thin, 1½″ diameter | 6 |
| Flour | 2½ tablespoons |
| Beans, cooked or dry, lima, navy, split | |
|     peas, cowpeas | ½ cup |
| baked beans, no pork | ¼ cup |
| Corn | ⅓ cup |
| Popcorn | 1 cup |
| Parsnips | ⅔ cup |
| Potatoes, white | 1 small |
| Potatoes, white, mashed | ½ cup |
| Potatoes, sweet | ¼ cup |
| Sponge cake, plain, 1½″ cube | 1 |
| Ice cream | ½ cup |
| Wine, red or white; any hard liquor | 4 ounces |
| Non-diet carbonated beverages | 6 ounces |

1. Check the foods listed next that are *not* on the Bread Exchange Equivalents list:

Cream

Cabbage

Pork chops

☐ Spaghetti
☐ Cream
☐ Cabbage
☐ Potatoes
☐ Pork chops
☐ Ice cream

2. Here is a list of foods from the bread exchange list. Write in the

amounts necessary to make these foods equal to one bread exchange.

_____ Baker beans, no pork

_____ Oyster crackers

_____ Corn flakes

_____ Popcorn

_____ Mashed white potatoes

_____ Ice cream

_____ Muffin, 2″ diameter

3. A soup recipe calls for:

½ cup navy beans
½ cup macaroni noodles
2½ tablespoons flour

How many bread exchanges will I need to make this soup?

_____ bread exchanges.

4. You are allowed 28 bread exchanges a week. If you wanted to eat an equal number of bread exchanges for each day of the week you would eat _____ bread exchanges a day. If you wanted to eat all of your exchanges for the week in slices of bread you would eat

3

4

28                    _____ slices of bread for the whole week.

5.  Circle the number of bread exchanges that you are allowed weekly on this plan:

28                    .  16       20       28       14

6.  If you eat ice cream (½ cup) for one bread exchange you must give up 2 fat exchanges. You already know that you are allowed to have 14 fat exchanges a week. Suppose you have arranged your fat exchanges so that you eat an equal number of fat exchanges each day.

2                     This gives you a total of _____ fat exchanges per day. If you ate ½ cup of ice cream on one day of the week, and you did not wish to exceed your self-imposed limitation of 2 daily fat exchanges, you would probably:

a.  Use 2 more fat exchanges any way.

b.  Use no more        b.  Use no more fat exchanges, be-
    fat exchanges          cause you already used 2 in the
                           ice cream.

2

7. When you eat ½ cup of ice cream, then, you must give up eating _____ fat exchanges.

8. The foods on the Bread Exchange Equivalents list that can be cooked should be measured *after* they are cooked. When you measure out a portion of popcorn for yourself, for example, you measure out 1 cup:

a. after

a. after it has been popped.
b. before it has been popped.

Stay as close to 9 meat exchanges daily as possible.

## MEAT EXCHANGES

| 1st Day | 2nd Day | 3rd Day | 4th Day | 5th Day | 6th Day | 7th Day |
|---|---|---|---|---|---|---|
| | | | | | | |
| | | | | | | |
| | | | | | | |
| | | | | | | |
| | | | | | | |
| | | | | | | |
| | | | | | | |

TOTALS

192

You are allowed 1 cup cooked vegetable A's per meal per day.

---

### COOKED VEGETABLE A EXCHANGES

| 1st Day | 2nd Day | 3rd Day | 4th Day | 5th Day | 6th Day | 7th Day |
|---------|---------|---------|---------|---------|---------|---------|
|  |  |  |  |  |  |  |
|  |  |  |  |  |  |  |
| **TOTALS** |  |  |  |  |  |  |
|  |  |  |  |  |  |  |

You are allowed a total of 14 fruit exchanges, so stay as close to 2 exchanges a day as possible.

---

### FRUIT EXCHANGES

| 1st Day | 2nd Day | 3rd Day | 4th Day | 5th Day | 6th Day | 7th Day |
|---------|---------|---------|---------|---------|---------|---------|
|  |  |  |  |  |  |  |
|  |  |  |  |  |  |  |
| **TOTALS** |  |  |  |  |  |  |
|  |  |  |  |  |  |  |

You are allowed a total of 7 Vegetable B exchanges a week, so keep the amounts you eat as close to 1 exchange daily as possible.

193

## VEGETABLE B EXCHANGES

*1st Day*　*2nd Day*　*3rd Day*　*4th Day*　*5th Day*　*6th Day*　*7th Day*

TOTALS

You are allowed a total of 14 fat exchanges for the entire week, so keep your daily consumption as close to 2 exchanges as possible.

## FAT EXCHANGES

*1st Day*　*2nd Day*　*3rd Day*　*4th Day*　*5th Day*　*6th Day*　*7th Day*

TOTALS

You are allowed a total of 7 milk exchanges weekly, so keep your daily consumption as close to 1 exchange as possible.

## MILK EXCHANGES

*1st Day  2nd Day  3rd Day  4th Day  5th Day  6th Day  7th Day*

TOTALS

Record the number of bread exchanges that you eat each day during the coming week in the spaces provided. You are allowed a total of 28 bread exchanges weekly, so keep your daily consumption as close to 4 as possible. Total each day as you go along.

## BREAD EXCHANGES

*1st Day  2nd Day  3rd Day  4th Day  5th Day  6th Day  7th Day*

TOTALS

This week the total number of grams of carbohydrates, proteins, and fats per exchange eaten are (per day):

|  | Carbohydrates | Proteins | Fats |
|---|---|---|---|
| Meat (9 per day) | 0 | 63 | 45 |
| Vegetable A's | 0 | 0 | 0 |
| Fruit (2 per day) | 20 | 0 | 0 |
| Vegetable B's | | | |
| (1 per day) | 7 | 2 | 0 |
| Fat (2 per day) | 0 | 0 | 10 |
| Milk (1 per day) | 12 | 8 | 10 |
| Bread (4 per day) | 60 | 8 | 0 |
| TOTAL GRAMS: | 99 | 81 | 65 |
| TOTAL CALORIES: | 396 | 324 | 585 = 1305 per day |

## WEEK SEVEN EXERCISE

This week most of you will reach your final goal:

BIKERS:    6 miles in 24 minutes
WALKERS:  4 miles in 60 minutes

This is the amount of daily exercise you will do every day for the rest of your life, even after you eventually reach your ideal weight and give up the diet.

If you do not reach this goal by the end of Week Seven, you will simply continue testing yourself and progressing at your own pace until you *do* reach it. You can stick with it on your own. By now you've become accustomed to exercising; you've seen it become an everyday

196

part of your life. But even more important, Week Seven is the time most of my patients—regardless of how close they are to the Week Seven goal—become exercise addicts.

No one was ever more recalcitrant about exercise— and ultimately more enthusiastic—than one of my favorite patients, Barbara. A former model who had put on over 50 pounds, Barbara wanted to be skinny again but fought the exercise program in every way. She faked it, tried to joke her way out of it, even lied about it. A patient at the clinic for almost a year, she was heavier at the end of that time than when she started.

Finally I decided on drastic action. I threatened to throw her out of the program if she did not appear at the office every day, exercise in front of witnesses, and let me feel her sweating forehead and rapid pulse at the end of each session. To my surprise and delight, she agreed. At the end of forty-nine days she had lost 33 pounds and loved exercising. A year later I met her at a party and was even more delighted. She had lost 55 pounds and was back to the weight and figure that had made her a success- ful model. She kept her stationary bicycle in the basement and exercised 24 minutes every night—without fail. In fact, she said, laughing, her date for that evening had arrived early, so she left him in her living room with a drink while she disappeared into the cellar for 24 minutes. "Can you picture it?" she said. "Me, the original Jewish princess, running past my date in a sweatsuit, dripping with perspiration! But I love my exercise, and I just refuse to give it up."

Are you beginning to feel the way Barbara does? The good feelings exercise gives you—increased energy, the relaxed feeling of health and well-being—should keep you working not just until you reach the Week Seven goal but permanently.

## WEEK SEVEN PROBLEMS

This is goody week. You can eat bread, candy, doughnuts, or spaghetti, and even have a cocktail.

This is also the week when many patients stop losing weight. Some even begin to gain.

Week Seven will not be discouraging for you if you understand what is happening to your body. Bread exchanges are mainly carbohydrate, plus a little protein. If they aren't burned off in your body, carbohydrates not only convert to fat, but also help your body retain water. That is why one unfortunate gentleman, famous in scientific literature, gained 18 pounds after one 4,000-calorie, high-carbohydrate meal. And, as you know, I gained eight pounds after eating one pizza.

But I don't gain weight like that anymore, even after binges. Even though my body is particularly susceptible to weight gain from carbohydrates, my physical condition prevents the enormous water gains that once victimized me so. Right now you too are developing that kind of efficiency in handling carbohydrates. But you're still only on the way. After six weeks of physical activity sessions, your physical condition is markedly improved. But most likely you are still not yet able to handle carbohydrates as efficiently as you will if you continue to exercise.

To find out how close you are to handling carbohydrates efficiently, I suggest that you eat all the food allowed in Week Seven. Weigh yourself daily for five days. If your weight loss continues to be steady, congratulations! You are using carbohydrates instead of storing them. Continue eating all the bread exchanges Week Seven allows.

If, at the end of the week, your weight loss stalls, cut back to one bread exchange per day. Finally, if you still have an unmoving scale, cut out the bread exchanges entirely. Spend an extra week on the Week Six diet, then reintroduce some bread exchanges into your menu.

Be patient. Continue your physical activity. Continue the Week Six diet, but test your progress by eating a few bread exchanges at least one day per week.

Carbohydrates are the primary cause of weight gain. If they prove troublesome for you, this means that your system tends to store carbohydrates rather than use the energy they provide. This has probably been your basic difficulty for all of your fat life. It certainly was mine.

If carbohydrates *are* the root of your problem, it may take as long as six months—and many physical-activity sessions—before your body adjusts to carbohydrates. But your body *can* change, and it *will* change if you work at it. Look at it this way: in return for a couple of months' work, I will be able to eat and drink whatever I please—*without* being reprimanded by my scale the next morning. Isn't a lifetime of carefree eating worth that much effort?

Have you reached your ideal weight? If yes, congratulations! If no, then this week you must decide what your ultimate goal is, and how fast you want to get there. When you've completed Week Seven, you can return to the Week Five diet (no bread or milk) if you want to lose more weight very quickly.

But remember that even if you eat all the exchanges allowed in Week Seven, your daily intake is still only 1,305 calories. With increased physical activity, this diet should allow you to continue losing weight. If your body indicates that you are able to eat from the bread group at the end of Week Seven (because you still register a steady weight loss), I'd suggest that you work toward your eventual goal slowly but pleasantly by eating all the Week Seven exchanges.

In the next chapter we'll talk more fully about where to go after the forty-nine days. For now, just review what you've learned from the test diet. Did fruit cause hunger pangs? Did milk produce unpleasant symptoms? Did bread bushwhack your weight losses? If so, did you drop any of these groups? If you have gone without any of these foods for several weeks, try reintroducing them now and note their effect. All of this information is necessary for you to devise a diet you can use most effectively until you've achieved your weight-loss goal.

Looking back over the last seven weeks, you'll recall that Week One presented a major difficulty—introducing physical activity into your life. Week Two, with its meat and vegetable A exchanges, probably gave you a gratifying weight loss, and Week Three's fruit exchanges may have caused some hunger pangs. The vegetable B's of Week Four don't usually present problems, but you might have reached a discouraging plateau that week. Week Five is generally easy. For some Week Six's milk exchanges caused indigestion. The Week Seven bread exchanges may even have temporarily halted your weight loss.

By now you've become quite adept at monitoring your body's responses to food. You feel the wonderful effects of improved physical condition and, like my patient Barbara, are "hooked" on your activity periods.

I sincerely hope this has been a gratifying new adventure for you. You have come a long way, and you have every reason to be proud of your perseverance. You deserve your success.

But right now you would probably like to know where you should go from here. You have reached the end of the forty-nine days, but *not* the end of exercising and, most likely, not the end of weight loss. There are still many pounds you would like to lose, and the next two chapters will tell you how.

# Some Fancy Exchange Dieting

"Suppose I want to eat something that is not specifically mentioned on the exchange lists, such as a chocolate bar or a piece of cake. Can I fit something like that into my diet?"

The answer is yes, of course. If you have more weight to lose, simply continue on the Week Seven diet. However, thanks to the exchange system, after the forty-nine days you can eat anything you want on the Week Seven diet while continuing to lose weight. You simply need to know what kinds of foodstuffs are contained in a food, and in what quantities. Then you can convert those figures into the exchanges you are already familiar with.

The United States Department of Agriculture has compiled a very handy book called *Composition of Foods,* which supplies information on the distribution of fats, carbohydrates, and proteins in nearly every food imaginable.

If you plan to lose a lot more weight and therefore intend to stay on the Week Seven diet for some time, I strongly recommend that you buy *Composition of Foods* so that you can eat a widely-varied diet and continue to lose weight. The book is available for $2.00 from:

> *Superintendent of Documents*
> *U.S. Government Printing Office*
> *Washington, D.C.   20402*

or from the Government Printing Office in your city.

*Food Values of Portions Commonly Used,* by Charles Frederick Bowes and Helen Nichols Church ( J. B. Lippincott Co.), is a similar guide available at most bookstores.

On the next pages you will learn how to perform some more complicated exchanges so that you can add your favorite foods to your diet without gaining weight.

1.   To measure the amount of fats, carbohydrates, and proteins contained in any food, we use a unit called the gram. In 1 ounce there

are 28 grams. In 2 ounces there are

56 _____ grams.

28      2. One ounce contains _____ grams; ½ ounce contains 14 grams.

3. The abbreviation for the words "gram" and "grams" is gm. If we were to use this shortened form to write the number of grams in an

gm.      ounce, we would write 28 _____.

4. Circle the number of grams contained in one ounce.

28 gm.      12 gm.      28 gm.

         36 gm.      0 gm.

5. There are 16 ounces in 1 pound.

8      In ½ pound there are _____ ounces.

6. To determine how many ounces there are in ½ pound, you divide 16

2      by _____.

7. Circle the number of ounces in a pound:

16      8      15      12      16

16
4

8. There are _____ ounces in a pound, so there must be _____ ounces in ¼ pound.

9. Circle the number of ounces in ¼ pound:

4

3      6      14      4

10. When you see "¼ pound" called for in a recipe, you know that if you measure out _____ ounces you will satisfy the requirement of the recipe.

4

11. One-quarter pound is equal to 4 ounces. One-eighth of a pound (half of ¼) is equal to _____ ounces.

2

12. When you read 2 ounces written on the wrapper of a chocolate bar, you know that another way of expressing the weight of that candy bar is (circle one):

⅛ pound

½ pound      ¼ pound
⅛ pound

13. Match the fractions of pounds listed with the number of ounces contained in that fraction.

c. 8 ounces

d. 4 ounces

b. 2 ounces

½ pound _____ a. 6 ounces

¼ pound _____ b. 2 ounces

⅛ pound _____ c. 8 ounces

d. 4 ounces

14. If you want to find out how many ounces make ¼ pound, you divide 16 by 4. Similarly, if you know that 1 pound of a certain food contains 20 grams of protein and you need to know how many grams of protein are in ¼ pound (or 4 ounces), you also divide by _____.

4

15. There are 40 grams of carbohydrate in 1 pound of a certain food. How many grams of carbohydrate would there be in ¼ pound?

10

8       10       20       40

16. If you want to know how many ounces make ⅛ pound you divide 16 by 8. Similarly, if you know that a certain food contains

32 grams of fat to the pound and you want to know how many grams of fat there are in ⅛ pound (2 ounces), you also divide by _____.

8

17. There are 40 grams of protein contained in a certain food, but you need to know how many grams of protein are contained in ⅛ pound of that food. In order to find out you would:

a. Divide 16 by 8.
b. Multiply 40 by 8.
c. Divide 40 by 8.
d. Guess

c. Divide 40 by 8

Study the following information.
One pound of sweet chocolate contains:
   20 grams protein
   159.2 grams fat
   262.6 grams carbohydrate

1. Which of the following contains 20 grams protein, 159.2 grams fat, and 262.6 grams carbohydrate? Underline one.

c. 1 pound of
sweet
chocolate

a. 100 grams of sweet chocolate.
b. ½ pound of sweet chocolate.
c. 1 pound of sweet chocolate.

2. To simplify, round off the numbers to eliminate fractions. Say that the grams of the basic foodstuffs contained in 1 pound of sweet chocolate are:

☐   20 grams protein
☐  160 grams fat
☐  262 grams  carbohydrate

10 gm. protein
80 gm. fat
131 gm. carbo-
hydrate

Now divide by 2 to find out how many grams of each foodstuff are contained in ½ pound of chocolate.

You found out how many grams of the three basic foodstuffs are contained in ½ pound of sweet chocolate by dividing the numbers of grams of the three basic foodstuffs contained in a full pound by 2. Similarly, if you wanted to know how many grams of the three foodstuffs are contained in ¼ pound of chocolate, you would divide the numbers of grams of each foodstuff contained in a pound of chocolate by 4.

Listed here are the amounts of the three foodstuffs contained in 1 pound of sweet chocolate. Divide by 4 to find the amounts contained in ¼ pound of sweet chocolate.

| | |
|---|---|
| 5 gm. protein | ☐ 20 grams protein |
| 40 gm. fat | ☐ 160 grams fat |
| 65½ gm. carbo-<br>hydrate | ☐ 262 grams carbohydrate |

You can find the amounts of the three basic foodstuffs contained in ⅛ pound (2 ounces) of sweet chocolate by dividing by 8. Here are the amounts of the three basic foodstuffs contained in 1 pound of sweet chocolate. Divide by 8 to find the number of grams of each foodstuff contained in ⅛ pound of sweet chocolate.

| | |
|---|---|
| 2.5 gm. protein | ☐ 20 grams protein |
| 20 gm. fat | ☐ 160 grams fat |

32.75 gm. carbo-          ☐  262 grams carbohydrate
   hydrate

You learned that ⅛ pound (2 ounces) of sweet chocolate contains:

2.5 grams of protein
20 grams of fat
32.75 grams of carbohydrate

Since we are only seeking to establish rough equivalents, let's round these numbers off again to make them easier to work with. Let's say that 2 ounces of sweet chocolate contains:

☐  3 grams protein
☐  20 grams fat
☐  33 grams carbohydrate

You know that one bread exchange contains 2 grams of protein and 15 grams of carbohydrate. If we subtract 2 bread exchanges from our diet on the day that we want to have the 2 ounces of sweet chocolate, we neatly cancel out all of the protein contained in the chocolate with 1 gram to spare, and all but 3 grams of the carbohydrate. After we subtract the 2 bread exchanges, the chocolate bar's contents will be:

☐  0 grams protein
☐  20 grams fat
☐  3 grams carbohydrate

We still have to take care of the fats. One fat exchange contains 5 grams of fat, so if we subtract 4 fat exchanges, we have canceled out the fats as well. After subtracting the fat exchanges, the power of the sweet chocolate bar to cause a weight gain is considerably lessened, for the content of the three foodstuffs after the cancellation process now looks like this:

- ☐ 0 grams protein
- ☐ 0 grams fat
- ☐ 3 grams carbohydrate

If you're wondering what you're going to do about the 3 grams of carbohydrate that are left over, the answer is, nothing. Remember that we took off a total of 4 grams of protein when we subtracted the 2 bread exchanges from our diet, so the calories contained in that extra gram of protein we gave up cancels out the calories contained in one of those renegade grams of carbohydrate (protein and carbohydrate both contain 4 calories to the gram). The amount of calories contained in the 2 remaining grams of carbohydrate (8 calories) is insignificant.

Perhaps you're troubled because you used up 4 fat exchanges in order to equal the 20 grams of fat contained in the chocolate. Previously I advised you not to exceed 2 fat exchanges a day. It *is* true that you should eat only 2 fat exchanges a day, but it is also true that you can have 4 fat exchanges a day if you use *skim milk* for your daily milk exchange. So, if you should ever want to use more than 2 fat exchanges a day, look to your milk exchanges to solve the dilemma.

There is another way to convert the 2 ounces of sweet chocolate into the food exchange equivalents that you are familiar with from this program. These are the foodstuffs contained in 2 ounces of sweet chocolate:

☐   3 grams protein
☐  20 grams fat
☐  33 grams carbohydrate

You know that one milk exchange contains 8 grams protein, 10 grams fat, and 12 grams carbohydrate. Let's subtract one half of a milk exchange from the foodstuff makeup of a sweet chocolate bar. One half of a milk exchange contains the following amounts of the three basic foodstuffs:

☐   4 grams protein
☐   5 grams fat
☐   6 grams carbohydrate

Subtracting ½ milk exchange from our menu plan on the day when we intend to eat the sweet chocolate bar leaves the amount of damage done looking like this:

☐   0 grams protein
☐  15 grams fat
☐  27 grams carbohydrate

We can easily eliminate that outstanding carbohydrate by deleting 3 fruit exchanges from our menu plan over the next two days (1 fruit exchange equals 10 grams carbohydrate), so that the remaining foodstuffs are as follows:

☐    0 grams protein
☐    15 grams fat
☐    0 grams carbohydrate

Now for the fats. To nullify the 15 grams of fat in the chocolate, delete your daily allowance of 2 fat exchanges (one fat exchange equals 10 grams fat), and make sure that the ½ milk exchange is consumed in skim milk products only. The reason for this is the fact that one whole milk exchange contains 10 grams of fat while ½ milk exchange contains 5 grams of fat, or exactly the amount you need to subtract from your menu plan on "sweet chocolate day."

As you work with numbers of grams of the basic foodstuffs, remember that it is not necessary to find exact correlations between the makeup of the foods you want to eat and the exchanges that you have been working with throughout the program. Rough approximations are good enough. If you happen to go over or under by a few grams of this or that or if the numbers of calories aren't exactly equal, don't worry about it. Nothing is amiss. You'll get better and better at making fast calculations

214

as you go along, and soon it will be second nature to you.

Remember, however, that the different foods that you may eat on the maintenance diet will cost you certain other foods from your exchange allowances, so weigh your priorities carefully. Before you eat a piece of fudge or a chocolate bar, think about the foods you're going to give up in order to stay within the diet and indulge yourself too. Then, if you absolutely must have it—go ahead.

There are also a lot of exchanges you can make without a great deal of arithmetic. For instance, if your job requires that you attend many business lunches, you might try exchanging a nice cold glass of dry white wine for a highball with lunch. A 4-ounce glass of wine equals one bread exchange, so you could have up to 16 ounces of wine per day and stay within the bounds of the diet. This is no more than most people would drink during a business luncheon.

Two glasses of white wine would use only two bread exchanges, but two highballs would use all your bread exchanges for the day (two for the whiskey, two for the ginger ale).

As you become more and more familiar with exchanging, eventually you will know in a flash what substitutions are possible, what foods to take from a buffet table. You will no longer be the deprived dieter who tries to nibble discreetly at a piece of Melba toast while the partygoers around you line hors-d'oeuvres up their arms and start eating from the shoulder down. Isn't that what everyone *seems* to be doing when you're limited to one cracker every six hours?

# After Forty-nine Days

You have now graduated from the forty-nine-day program. During the last seven weeks you have worked hard to (1) test your body's reactions to various food groups; (2) learn the fundamentals of exchange dieting; (3) begin a regular physical-fitness program. You learned a lot about losing weight, and about why you *gain* weight.

It's been tough, but I'm sure you feel it's been worth it.

Now it's time to create a new plan, based on your own experiences during the last seven weeks, which you can carry on with for as long as necessary. This plan will enable you to keep your weight under control easily, free of the tyranny of paying meticulous attention to food intake and without the fear of recurring overweight.

How you proceed now depends on your weight-loss goal, but no matter what diet you decide to follow, you should be continuing your exercise periods *without fail. If you have already achieved the Week Seven goal* (for bikers, 6 miles in 24 minutes; for walkers, 4 miles in 60 minutes), you have achieved minimal physical fitness. As you look back, I'll bet you can't believe how much you've improved your performance in just seven weeks. Now set yourself a new goal: maximal fitness. Instead of exercising every six days and resting on the seventh, go to seven exercise periods a week. You are still creating lean body mass, working for the day when you need so many calories to maintain body weight that you can return to normal eating.

*If you have not yet achieved the Week Seven goal,* don't be distressed. Remember: to become physically fit your body must complete an enormous reconstruction job. The whole process may take a few more months, so *don't rush.* Just continue doing the best you can *every day* and don't start going easy on yourself. Keep on testing to see whether you can't go just a bit further than you did yesterday. If you stick with daily exercise, your body *will* respond and you *will* succeed.

❖     ❖     ❖

Your diet from now on will be determined by your own weight goal. *If you haven't achieved fitness and still have more weight to lose,* you may continue on the Week Seven diet for as long as you like; unlike Weeks One and Two, Week Seven's diet is nutritionally complete and safe for a long-term diet. There are 1,305 calories in Week Seven, and while you are losing weight you should also be completely satisfied with what you are eating.

Or you may wish to return to the Week Five diet. Although nutritionally complete, it lacks the milk and bread exchanges of Weeks Six and Seven. This means that it is less filling, but if you have the willpower it will mean quicker weight loss. And, of course, the Week Five diet is best for those of you whose weight loss halted when the bread group was introduced into the test diet.

No matter which diet you choose, keep in mind the results of your test diet. If you had to eliminate any exchanges during the seven weeks, every so often try reintroducing those foods. Continued exercise will eventually enable you to absorb the sugars in fruit or the carbohydrates in bread, so test yourself occasionally. Try adding half the exchanges you eliminated and see what happens. If you continue to lose weight, you've strengthened your body to the point where it can absorb the quick sugar in fruit successfully, leaving nothing to store as fat. Once you've reached that point, you can start eating all of your daily fruit exchanges. The same is true if you leave out bread or milk. Try reintroducing them and see what happens.

*If you have achieved minimal fitness, but still want to lose more weight,* stick with the Week Seven diet. Meanwhile, if Week Seven's diet leaves you hungry, you can begin adding some additional food to your daily intake. Try eating two or three exchanges of any food group as a snack. That extra small meal will tend to make you less hungry during the day and, now that you're minimally fit, shouldn't put any weight on.

Snack like this for a week, then check your weight. If it is still going down, add a few more exchanges to the Week Seven diet. You might begin by increasing all exchanges by 25 percent—eleven meat exchanges instead of nine; one more bread and one more fat or fruit exchange per day. After a week on the increased exchange diet, check yourself again. Is your weight still going down?

If so, increase your exchanges by 50 percent—thirteen meats; three fruits, three fats, six breads, and one more vegetable B or milk exchange. Has your weight loss stopped? Maybe you should drop back to a 25 percent increase in exchanges, or even go all the way back to the Week Seven diet, if you are anxious to speed up your weight loss again.

*If you've achieved minimal fitness* and *lost all the weight you desire,* gradually return to normal eating while continuing the exercise schedule. One way you can judge whether you've created significantly more LBM is to test your body's response to troublesome foods. Have you reintroduced whatever exchanges you dropped during the test diet? Until you can safely eat *all* the food groups, you should continue to be cautious. In the meantime, you can snack on additional exchanges and, if no weight gain occurs, add more and more exchanges to the Week Seven diet, using the method explained above.

Patients often wonder what the effects of a food binge would be, now that they are past the forty-nine days. If you've achieved minimal fitness, a binge won't do much damage. Simply return to the basic Week Seven diet, and within a few days your body will dispose of the overdose of carbohydrates and fats. If you *aren't* fit, forego all bingeing till you are!

Regardless of whether you are fit or not, as thin as you wish or not—how do you *feel?* I hope your answer is "Terrific!" Now that the forty-nine days are over, do you feel different about food? It probably seems just as delicious as ever, but a bit less important than when you began the test diet. If so, physical activity has given you a more normal appetite, so you eat when you're hungry instead of when you have nothing else to do.

At this moment you are closer than you have been for years to being permanently slim. Together we have worked through the most difficult time—the beginning of physical activity. Now you are well on your way. If you stay with your diet (temporarily) and your exercise (permanently), you will soon feel even more energetic, slim, and *alive* than you do now.

Won't it be nice when only your closest friends (and your tailor) remember that you used to be fat?

No matter how fat you may still think you are, inside you are becoming a thin person. Your body is beginning to function as if it were thin and soon your mind will have no choice but to agree.

You are about to begin a new kind of life. What will it be like? Well, judging by my own experience, it will be marvelous. Looking thin and feeling full of energy has improved my self-image enormously. I'm much more confident in my work, and I *should* be—now that I'm healthier and more energetic, I work better. One day last week I flew to Los Angeles from my home in San Francisco, spent eight hours in conference there, prepared my income tax returns, and in general withstood more aggravation than any man should have to bear within a twenty-four-hour period. Five years ago the frustrations of that day would have killed me. Now I am capable of tolerating a lot more stress, and my twenty-four minutes of daily exercise acts as a natural, normal tranquilizer. At eight that night I climbed on a friend's stationary bike and rode six miles in twenty-four minutes. Immediately afterward I felt refreshed and relaxed enough to walk a mile and a half to the Century Plaza Hotel for one of their delicious hot fudge brownies.

You'll also feel much younger in your new life. Once again you will bounce up stairs instead of waiting for an elevator. You'll walk to the supermarket rather than go through the hassle of getting the car out of the garage, driving a few blocks, then hunting for a parking space. When the ski season starts, your body won't ache after the first day's workout. You'll tear around the tennis court without worrying about your heart. In my scuba diving course I've discovered that I can keep up with the eighteen-year-olds in the class. I'm thirty-nine years old, working at least ten hours a day, fighting the American rat race, but I feel as if I'm twenty-four and coasting.

Best of all, in your new life you will be able to enjoy food without fearing it, or being obsessed by it. I don't worry about my weight, and my eating habits show it. It's not at all unusual for me to begin the day with an enormous breakfast of pancakes with butter and syrup, sausages and cheese. In the middle of the morning I'll snack, usually on some big carbohydrate bomb like chocolate-covered cookies. Even if I'm not hungry at lunchtime I will most likely have a social or business lunch where I'll put away a roll with butter and a large chef's salad, smothered in dressing. My wife loves to cook, and when I get home at night I can count on another big meal. By the end of the day I have racked up at least 4,000 calories. Yet I know that by the next morning my weight will be about the same as it was *before* those 4,000 calories. It's wonderful to feel impervious to calories, and marvelous not to be preoccupied with weight.

The only real *problem* with exercise is that soon you no longer have a diet to talk about.

# Final Thoughts

It wouldn't be honest of me to end this book without a word to those of you who tried and didn't make it. Perhaps you walked for a few days. Then your muscles felt stiff and you decided to give them a rest—permanently. Or you stuck with the diet beautifully, but then your husband's birthday came up and the children baked him a cake . . . and the next day you knew your scale would register no loss . . . so with your coffee you had one of the doughnuts you'd bought for the kids. And that was that.

My patients have had spectacular results with this plan, but of course I've witnessed some failures. Some people make it all the way through Week Seven but fall apart once they're on their own. Every single failure bothers me. I've seen people come to the plan with joy and enthusiasm, watched them progress, work vigorously, diet honestly . . . and come back to my clinic six months later, faces once again swollen with fat.

Even if you are now thirty pounds lighter than when you opened this book, you have to be aware that you will always be capable of becoming a fat person again. Now that you are physically fit it will be harder for you to gain weight; it will take longer. But your body still has all its hereditary and hormonal potential to revert to the fat, out-of-shape condition it was in just a short time ago. When I was struggling through the first forty-nine days of diet and exercise, I often thought to myself, "What's the use? This is the twentieth century; it's absurd to work up a sweat and deprive myself of food. Why not enjoy what this century has to offer and resign myself to the fat life circumstances seem to have decreed?"

Nevertheless, I eventually chose to fight my natural tendency toward obesity. I had a lot of reasons. For one thing, I am vain and I like to feel that I'm attractive to others. I have a wonderful wife and I want to see my daughters grow up. I want to experience everything this world has to offer, and for that I need the energy that comes with a thirty-four inch waist.

You know what I'm talking about. Think about how terrific you look—hasn't everyone told you so? When you catch sight of your reflection in shopwindows, don't you feel excited instead of depressed? Some of the joys of thin life are small ones—like being able to crowd into the bucket seat of a compact car with two other people . . . or bending over to retrieve something without bashing into your own stomach.

I am so delighted with my life and my personal appearance that I will never let the goals I've achieved slip away. If I know I've eaten more carbohydrates than I should have today, I exercise harder tomorrow and I don't look upon that exercise as punishment for wickedness. It is simply a very small price to pay for a wonderful life. Diabetics give themselves insulin shots; former alcoholics stay away from liquor; I exercise. In the larger scheme of things, I don't feel it's such a terrible burden to bear.

If you didn't succeed this time, do me this favor. Don't rush out for another diet book a friend just told you about. You've bought the last fat book you'll ever need. It's honest, it's workable, it's safe, and when you are ready to succeed, it will tell you how. Put this book on the shelf. Wait awhile and try again. I failed four times on the stationary bicycle before I finally got back on and rode into this new world.

I swear, the flowers here smell better, the sun shines brighter, the lovemaking is sweeter, the laughter is happier. Please join me. Being slim and fit is really *living*.

# Week One Recipes

The recipes that follow are basic, simple suggestions for making your food look and taste interesting during Week One.

Remember: use a Teflon frying pan—to avoid cooking with fat—and an ovenproof baking dish whenever possible.

Specific brands are mentioned only when they are reliably very low-calorie.

Each of these recipes will serve one.

A    EGG WITH MUSHROOM FILLING

*1 small mushroom, finely chopped*
*1 sprig fresh parsley, finely chopped*

*oregano, thyme, or rosemary*
*2 teaspoons beef bouillon*
*1 egg, beaten*

Sauté mushroom, parsley, and herbs in beef bouillon over low heat for 1 to 2 minutes. Add egg and cook over higher heat until done.

B    **GRAPEFRUIT**

Sprinkle half grapefruit with cinnamon and heat in 350° F oven for 10 minutes. Section grapefruit and serve hot.

C    **RUFFLED SALAD**

*lettuce*
*1 thinly sliced cucumber*

Toss lettuce and cucumber with lemon juice or Good Seasons Lo-Calorie Dressing, or Zero Salad Dressing.

**ZERO SALAD DRESSING**

*½ cup tomato sauce*
*2 tablespoons lemon juice or vinegar*
*1 tablespoon finely chopped onion*
*salt and pepper*
*chopped parsley, green pepper, horseradish,*
    *mustard, if desired*

Combine ingredients and shake well.

D    CHICKEN IMPERIAL

*6 ounces chicken broth*
*2 teaspoons Worcestershire sauce*
*garlic powder*
*curry powder*
*dry mustard*
*paprika*
*Tabasco sauce (optional)*
*1 8-ounce chicken breast*

Preheat oven to 350° F. In a small saucepan, combine chicken broth and Worcestershire sauce. Sprinkle garlic powder, curry powder, dry mustard, paprika, Tabasco sauce to taste. Blend ingredients over low heat for 5 minutes.

Roast chicken skin side up for 1 hour, basting with sauce every 15 minutes. Serve.

E    BROCCOLI ITALIENNE

*¾ cup broccoli*
*1 clove garlic*
*1 tablespoon chicken broth*
*oregano*
*1 teaspoon lemon juice*

Gently steam broccoli in ½ cup water. Drain. Sauté crushed garlic in chicken broth over low heat for 2 minutes. Add large pinch oregano and the lemon

juice. Remove crushed garlic clove. Pour over
drained broccoli and serve.

**F    EVE SALAD**

*1 apple, sectioned*
*¼ cup cottage cheese*
*lettuce*
*cinnamon*

Center cottage cheese on a lettuce leaf; arrange
sectioned apple around it. Dust cottage cheese with
cinnamon.

**G    MAGIC MUSHROOM SALAD**

*¾ cup fresh mushrooms, sliced*
*salad dressing*
*2 tablespoons finely sliced scallions*
*lettuce*

Marinate mushrooms and scallions in Zero Salad
Dressing. Serve over lettuce.

**H    STEAK PACIFICA**

*1 8-ounce steak*
*¼ cup Kikkoman Hawaiian Teriyaki Sauce*
*1 clove fresh garlic, sliced thin*
*ginger to taste*
*MSG ( optional )*
*¾ teaspoon lime juice*

Trim all fat off steak. Combine all other ingredients in a baking dish, then add meat. Marinate 1 hour or more, turning the meat frequently. Broil steak in a broiler or over charcoal until brown and glazed on each side but still rare inside. Serve.

I     LEMON GREEN BEANS

*1 tablespoon chicken broth*
*1 clove garlic, minced*
*1 tablespoon lemon juice*
*¾ cup green beans, cooked*

Sauté garlic in chicken broth and lemon juice. Pour over green beans and serve.

J     RIVIERA SALAD

*lettuce*
*tomato, cut in 6 wedges*
*Zero Salad Dressing or Good Seasons Lo-Calorie*
    *Salad Dressing*

Combine all ingredients.

**K    BAKED PERCH ITALIANO**

*8-ounce perch*
*1 small can marinara sauce (7¾ ounces)*
*1 fresh lemon*
*1 sprig fresh parsley*

Preheat oven to 375° F. Wash and dry the fish thoroughly. In baking dish, spoon 2 tablespoons marinara sauce over the fish. Bake for 25 minutes. Remove from the oven and pour the remaining sauce over the fish with the juice of half of the lemon. Replace fish in the oven and bake for 15 minutes. Top with parsley and thin slice of fresh lemon. Serve.

**L    BROILED HERB CHICKEN**

*1 clove fresh garlic*
*8-ounce chicken breast*
*soy sauce*
*thyme or tarragon*

Slice garlic in half, and rub the chicken with the inside of the garlic. Brush chicken with soy sauce, and sprinkle with ¼ teaspoon of thyme or tarragon. Place in broiler, skin side up, 6 inches below flame for 9 minutes. Turn the breast over and broil for another 9 minutes. Finally, turn the chicken skin side up again for 5 minutes. Serve at once. Or allow to cool, wrap in aluminum foil, and save for lunch.

M  SWEDISH SPINACH

*½ cup spinach*
*MSG (optional)*
*¼ teaspoon nutmeg*

Cook and drain spinach. Add seasonings to spinach while hot, then serve.

N  TOMATO À LA RUSSE

*3 lettuce leaves*
*1 tomato, whole*
*¼ cup cottage cheese*

Arrange lettuce leaves on a plate. Hold tomato over flame on a wooden-handled fork until skin pops and can be peeled away. Slice "lid" off top of tomato. Scoop pulp out of the center and remove seeds. Mash the pulp with the cottage cheese. Stuff the tomato shell with this mixture and serve.

O  BEEF STROGANOFF

*8-ounce steak, cut into ¼-inch strips*
*3 tablespoons beef consommé*

1 teaspoon prepared mustard
dillweed

Sauté steak strips over medium heat in the consommé until well browned. Add mustard to the
sauce in the frying pan with the steak. Simmer 3
minutes. Sprinkle a pinch of dillweed over the meat
and serve.

P    STUFFED MUSHROOMS

½ cup fresh mushrooms
¼ cup spinach, cooked and drained
Salt and pepper

Separate stems gently from mushroom caps. Chop
stems with the spinach. Season with salt and pepper
to taste. Fill the mushroom caps with a small mound
of the spinach and mushroom mixture. Bake the
mushrooms in an aluminum-foil envelope in a 350°
F oven until they are hot and serve.

Q    SUNSHINE SALAD

lettuce
segments from ½ grapefruit
Zero Salad Dressing or Good Seasons Lo-Calorie
    Salad Dressing

Combine all ingredients.

**R  CHICKEN ROSEMARY**

*8-ounce chicken breast*
*chicken broth*

*powdered rosemary*

Preheat broiler. Brush the chicken with the broth and place it skin side up in a baking dish 6 inches below flame for 9 minutes. Turn breast over and broil for another 9 minutes. Turn the chicken again, sprinkle with rosemary, and cook 5 minutes. Serve, or allow to cool, and wrap in foil for lunch.

**S  SNOWDRIFT SALAD**

*½ cup cauliflower flowerets, cooked and chilled*
*Zero Salad Dressing or Good Seasons Lo-Calorie*
    *Salad Dressing*
*1 slice Melba toast, crushed*
*lettuce leaves*

Dip the cauliflower in the salad dressing and then into the Melba-toast crumbs. Serve on lettuce leaves.

**T  EGG WITH TOMATO**

*1 tomato slice, ¼-inch thick, cubed*
*1 sprig parsley, finely chopped*
*pinch of basil*
*pinch of onion powder*

237

2 *teaspoons beef bouillon*
1 *egg, beaten*

Sauté tomato cubes, parsley, basil, and onion powder in beef bouillon. Increase heat, add egg. Mix well and serve.

**U    HICKORY STEAK**

*8-ounce steak*
*onion powder*
*MSG (optional)*
*black pepper, freshly ground*
*hickory-smoke salt*

Sprinkle steak on both sides with seasonings and let stand for 1 hour. Broil. Serve hot, or allow to cool and wrap in aluminum foil for lunch.

**V    TOMATO PROVENÇALE**

*tomato*
*basil*
*thyme*

Peel tomato over open flame (see recipe N). Slice the tomato in half horizontally. Sprinkle each half with basil and thyme. Broil until hot and bubbly.

**W   EGG WITH ZUCCHINI**

*small can chopped zucchini*
*oregano or thyme*
*2 teaspoons beef bouillon*
*1 egg, beaten*

Sauté 1 heaping teaspoon zucchini with a pinch of oregano or thyme in bouillon over low heat. Increase heat, add beaten egg. Mix well and serve.

**X   EMERALD SALAD**

*1 green pepper*
*lettuce leaves*
*Zero Salad Dressing or Good Seasons Lo-Calorie
    Salad Dressing*

Cut green pepper into ½-inch cubes. Mix with lettuce leaves. Add dressing to taste.

**Y   ORIENTAL CHICKEN SALAD**

*¼ cup soy sauce*
*2 teaspoons Worcestershire sauce*
*¼ teaspoon powdered ginger*
*¼ teaspoon garlic powder*
*8-ounce chicken breast, boned*
*onion powder*
*paprika*

*1 orange, separated into segments, with membrane removed*
*¾ cup lettuce*
*1 slice Melba toast*

Mix sauces and ginger and garlic powders, pour over the chicken breast. Allow to marinate several hours. Place chicken in aluminum foil for baking. Sprinkle with onion powder and paprika. Bake at 350° F for 20 minutes, or until browned and crisp. Allow chicken to cool. Cut chicken into ½-inch strips. Pour 2 tablespoons of sauce onto chicken strips. Mix well. Add orange segments. Mix again. Arrange the salad on lettuce. Crumble Melba toast and sprinkle crumbs over top.